Stuttering: Differential Evaluation and Therapy

HUGO H. GREGORY

D1564615

5341 Industrial Oaks Boulevard
Austin, Texas 78735

**The PRO-ED
studies in
communicative disorders**

Series editor
HARVEY HALPERN

Library of Congress Cataloging in Publication Data
Gregory, Hugo H.
  Stuttering : differential evaluation and therapy.

  (The PRO-ED studies in communicative disorders)
  Bibliography: p.
  1. Stuttering. 2. Speech therapy. I. Title.
II. Series.
RC424.G72   1986   616.85'54   86-490
ISBN 0-89079-093-0

5341 Industrial Oaks Boulevard
Austin, Texas 78735

10 9 8 7 6 5 4 3 2 1   86 87 88 89 90 91

Contents

Preface

This monograph describes a differential evaluation process derived from clinical observations and current research and then describes differential treatment strategies based on this evaluation. Prevention of stuttering and the management of early developmental stages are followed by a discussion of therapy for more confirmed upper school-age or adult secondary stutterers. Then it is shown how therapy for more confirmed stutterers of elementary school age draws on techniques used with the younger and older groups. Special topics included are parent counseling; more direct fluency-enhancing procedures for preschool children; the management of complicating speech, language, and behavior factors; and transfer and maintenance. The reader is given a concise description of the evaluation and treatment process for children and adults in a way that leads to the use of a problem-solving approach with individual subjects.

Stuttering: Differential Evaluation and Therapy

Introduction

Although there may be slight variations in definition, stuttering is a term used to indicate a type and quantity of disfluency not characteristic of the age and immediate speaking situation of the child. As we will see, it is better to consider beginning stuttering in terms of disfluency, as a dimensional problem in a child, not an either-or matter (Andrews et al., 1983). Stuttering seems to begin in childhood between the ages of 18 months and 9 years, mostly between 2 and 5 years of age. It is complex in its development, according to some recent data, and may, according to parent reports, either develop rather suddenly or over a period of weeks (Johnson et al., 1959; Yairi, 1983). Surveys (Bloodstein, 1981) reveal that stuttering is present in about 0.9% to 1.1% of the school-age population. It has long been recognized that the incidence of defective speech, whether on a functional or organic basis, is higher among males than females (Eisenson, 1965). The male-female ratio among stutterers as revealed by surveys (Bloodstein, 1981) has varied from 2.2:1 to 5.3:1 with evidence that the sex ratio increases with age. Either more boys begin to stutter later or girls tend to recover from stuttering more readily. Regarding recovery, about two thirds of children who show a noticeable degree of stuttering at some time dur-

1

ing their development regain normally fluent speech. This observation is based on retrospective research, clinical observations, and parent reports (Andrews & Harris, 1964; Cooper, 1972; Sheehan & Martyn, 1966, 1970). Finally, there appears to be a genetic factor that predisposes certain children to stuttering, but environmental factors are assumed to interact with genetic dispositions (Andrews & Harris, 1964; Howie, 1981; Kidd, 1980).

This problem of the fluency of speech has been studied extensively and, in the opinion of most speech pathologists, fruitfully during the last 50 years of an increasingly more experimental era in the behavioral sciences. Results of research have been conflicting at times (Bloodstein, 1981; Eisenson, 1965; Van Riper, 1982), possibly another demonstration of the complexity of stuttering or the heterogeneity of stutterers as a group. However, we do have more definitive descriptions of the behavior and factors associated with its variation (Bloodstein, 1981; Johnson, 1955), and we do know more about the differing characteristics of persons who stutter (Andrews et al., 1983). In addition, a better understanding of the development of stuttering (Gregory & Hill, 1980, 1984; Johnson et al., 1959; Riley & Riley, 1979, 1980; Wall & Myers, 1984) has led to optimism about our ability to prevent it or to reverse the tide of the developmental process at an early stage (Gregory, 1984a). There has been much progress in the techniques evaluating the results of stuttering therapy (Ingham, 1984; Perkins, 1979; Ryan, 1974, 1979) and in coming to terms with the problems involved in the persistence of improvement over time (Boberg, 1981; Fraser-Gruss, 1983). As will be discussed in the section on therapy, the need for specific transfer and maintenance activities has been recognized. Gains in understanding the nature of developing problems in children and chronic stuttering problems of older children and adults have led to significant improvements in evaluation and therapy.

Speech Fluency in Children

As language develops and as articulatory proficiency is acquired, there are at the same time changes in the flow of children's speech, noted mainly by the quality and quantity of speech disfluency. To establish a frame of reference for assessing a child's speech, the following statements provide a brief analysis and summary of our information about the fluency of children's speech.

1. *Frequency of disfluency.* Pauses, revisions, and interjections (nonrepetitious disfluencies) occur most frequently (Brownell, 1973; DeJoy, 1975; Wexler & Mysak, 1982). Part-word sound and syllable repetitions and pro-

longations of sounds are least frequent (Brownell, 1973; DeJoy, 1975; Haynes & Hood, 1977; Wexler & Mysak, 1982). Two-year-olds may show considerable part-word repetition; yet most studies indicate that this part-word repetition begins to decrease during the third year (Johnson, 1955; Yairi, 1981). When language is developing rapidly during the second and third years, single-syllable word repetitions are frequent at the beginning of syntactic units (Yairi, 1981). There is reasonably good evidence that disfluency, especially repetitious types, decreases generally following the third year (DeJoy, 1975; Wexler & Mysak, 1982). There is a rather large inter-subject and intrasubject variability (the latter based on repeated measures of disfluency types in the same child taken at 3- or 4-month intervals) (DeJoy, 1975; Gottfred, 1979; Haynes & Hood, 1977; Wexler & Mysak, 1982; Yairi, 1981, 1982). Yairi (1982) concludes: "Unlike several other aspects of speech and language such as sound acquisition, articulatory precision, and syntactic skills that usually assume a one-way developmental course, disfluency stands out as a phenomenon which is prone to alternating reversals" (p. 159).

2. *Situational differences.* Parent reports and clinical observations reveal these differences; however, research results have been equivocal (Johnson, 1942; Silverman, 1972). It appears that situational effects are highly individual. This is a problem in terms of research and should be taken into consideration in clinical evaluation.

3. *Grammatical effects.* In adults and school-age children research has shown that content words such as nouns, adjectives, and adverbs are stuttered more frequently (Brown, 1938). However, since content words tend to be longer words, and longer words are more frequently stuttered, the length factor may have a confounding influence (Taylor, 1966). Most studies of either nonstuttering or stuttering preschool children have revealed a greater than expected number of disfluencies on function words and pronouns at the beginning of syntactic units (Bloodstein & Gantwerk, 1967; Helmreich & Bloodstein, 1973; Silverman, 1973). Younger children probably respond to these syntactic units as the basic units of speech formulation and motor speech production. We need more research on the manner in which the transition increasingly occurs from more stuttering on function words to more on content words between the ages of 4 and 8.

4. *Sex differences.* Since there is a male-female ratio of about 4 to 1 among stutterers, it would be statistically neat to find a higher incidence of disfluency in male children. Studies (Davis, 1939; Oxtoby, 1943; Yairi, 1981) have tended to show a higher frequency of syllable repetition in boys, but no differences have been statistically significant. Recently Yairi (1981)

reported a trend for boys to show more repetitions per instance of syllable repetition.

5. *Listener reactions.* Studies have been done in which listeners judged samples of speech drawn from the speech of nonstuttering and stuttering children. These studies have shown that sound and syllable repetitions and disfluencies rated as severe are more often classified as stuttering than are revisions and interjections (Boehmler, 1958; Giolas & Williams, 1958; Williams & Kent, 1958).

6. *Speech of stutterers.* Early studies (Davis, 1939; Voelker, 1944) showed that speakers who are considered to be stutterers demonstrate a substantially greater frequency of sound and syllable repetitions and prolongations. In comparing male stuttering and nonstuttering children between the ages of 2 and 8, Johnson et al. (1959) reported that stuttering children showed significantly more sound and syllable repetition, word repetition, phrase repetition, broken words, and prolonged sounds. In the last of three studies of the onset and development of stuttering, Johnson et al. (1959) reported that the parents of stuttering children observed the presence of sound and syllable repetition at the onset of stuttering significantly more often than was reported by parents of a matched group of nonstuttering children.

There appears to be meaning in the finding that one-syllable word repetitions occur rather frequently in the speech of most children, but that breaks in fluency at the word level (sound and syllable repetitions and prolongations of sounds) occur less frequently in the speech of most children. When the latter types of disfluencies occur more frequently in a child's speech, we are more concerned. Increased concern is also supported by the observations that stuttering children show more of these disfluencies and that listeners are more likely to judge within-word disfluencies as characteristics of stuttering. A point made by Williams and Kent (1958) is that a child may become known as a stutterer because he or she repeats syllables. They warn that this could have an unfortunate effect on the child's speech if it meant an adverse reaction by listeners. I will say more about this as I define stuttering and later as I describe evaluation procedures.

Definition of Stuttering

When I was first a student it was easier to define stuttering. Now it is more complex and difficult. Perkins (1983) has recently discussed the problem of definition in commenting on a review of research findings or "facts" about stuttering by Andrews et al. (1983). Quite correctly Perkins points out, as have others, that our research is all influenced by the way in which we define stuttering and, based on this definition, choose subjects for study. Of course, clinical judgments are also based on our orienting definition.

A definition of stuttering has to take into consideration the age of the subject (with reference to cognitive, emotional, and social development), the types and frequency of disfluency, and the subject's attitude about speaking. If the definition is to relate to etiology, we have to make the best statement possible about the factors that appear to predispose a child to stuttering or contribute to the development of stuttering. The latter includes environmental factors.

For introductory purposes stuttering can be defined as a higher frequency of sound, syllable, and one-syllable word disfluency (more irregular in rhythm and averaging two to four repetitions per instance) and prolonged sounds or postures of the speech mechanism. There may be a disruption of air flow or phonation between repetitions, or a schwa-sounding vowel may be substituted for the correct one in the repetition of a syllable. There may be other signs of increased tension in the lips, jaw, larynx, or chest as well as accessory movements of bodily parts not closely associated with speaking. A covert feature of stuttering includes expectation of difficulty and frustration, which lead to avoidance and inhibitory behaviors — reactions that can be described by older children and adults and that may be mentioned by a preschool child. In the latter we can only assume that covert reactions accompany the development of overt behaviors and are more likely to be present the longer the problem exists. In keeping with the social nature of speaking, as stuttering persists, the person's self-concept is influenced by the speaking problem, and unadaptive attitudes develop.

PART ONE

Differential Evaluation of Children with Fluency Problems Including Stuttering

In this discussion, fluency problems including stuttering will be considered as the entire continuum of fluency deviation from minimal (about which there is some agreement but which may be perceived differently by different listeners) to the clearly evident struggling behavior of a severe stutterer.

The search for a cause has been characteristic of the historical interest in and study of stuttering. During the period after 1925, when speech pathology became more scientific and research-oriented in its search for the etiology of stuttering, many investigations were carried out in an attempt to find an organic, psychogenic, or psychologically learned origin in the disorder (Bloodstein, 1981; Van Riper, 1982). Many group studies involving statistical comparisons of stutterers and nonstutterers have been done.

Contradictory findings, or at least variations in findings, occurred often enough to encourage such ideas as "stutterers are a heterogeneous group," "there are different avenues to becoming a stutterer," or "contributing factors combine in various ways to produce stuttering." The point of view that will underline the ensuing consideration of differential evaluation is that various patterns of contributing factors (characteristic of the subject and environmental variables) can occasion more disfluency and possibly different types of disfluency and/or stuttering behavior. Certainly these factors should be evaluated and considered carefully in the treatment of an incipient or more advanced stuttering problem.

We may be uncertain about the specific cause of stuttering, but we do know that the manipulation of certain subject and environmental factors reduces it. Much successful treatment is based upon this premise. The following consideration of differential evaluation will give the rationale of certain procedures with reference to theoretical concepts and clinical or research findings about stuttering. These differential evaluation procedures will serve as a basis for a subsequent section on therapy.

The diagnostic evaluation is divided into three major parts: (1) informal observation, (2) case history, and (3) formal observation and testing. This introductory discussion will focus on children, leaving to the reader or the instructor the generalization of these procedures to teenagers and adults.

Informal Observation

Speech behavior and bodily tension, responses to changes in the examiner's manner, enjoyment of communication, and responses to parents and authority figures are all aspects of informal observation.

The evaluation process begins as the clinician meets the parents and the child for the first time. The child's speech is observed as well as the way in which the parents and the child interact. These brief observations serve as a guide when the clinician takes the case history and makes the more formal diagnostic evaluation. Referring to the continuum of disfluency from *More Usual* to *More Unusual* shown in Figure 1, the clinician considers whether the child seems to be emitting borderline atypical or atypical disfluencies to the extent that we should be concerned.

Continuing informal observations, the examiner varies his or her speaking rate, vocal inflection, and other aspects of manner to assess the way in which the subject's speech is a response to stimulus conditions in the environment. These responses are indicative of the social-psychological nature of the problem and the importance of environmental modification and desensitization procedures in therapy. Engaging the child in conversation, the examiner watches for signs of anger, frustration, withdrawal, and avoidance. Does the child seem to appreciate communication in spite of frustration or is the child realizing little reward from talking? If there are signs of the latter, the clinician may have to change this attitude to some degree very early in the therapy process before much else can be accomplished. The way in which certain stimulus conditions elicit stuttering can also be observed as the child interacts with the parents and other authority figures. In addition, I have found it beneficial to note the parents' speaking rates and the quantity and quality of disfluency in their speech. If the parents' rate is rapid, we may ask them to speak more calmly and slowly with the child. If there are signs that a parent is or has been a stutterer, he or she may be more sensitive to disfluency.

Case History

The case history includes information such as the informant's statement of the problem, any family history of stuttering, general developmental and medical factors, speech and language development, environmental conditions, and educational progress.

Informant's Statement of the Problem

Usually, in the examining situation, the parent or another informant has made a brief statement of the problem previous to the informal observation just described. However, this may be asked for again and reviewed at the beginning of the case history. It is interesting to note the way in which the parents and others perceive the problem in comparison with the clinician's observation and even with the child's own evaluation. For example, the parent may be quite disturbed about disfluencies that do not seem to the clinician to be of the quality or quantity to cause concern. Hopefully, there may be no indication that the child is reacting abnormally.

Johnson's listener-speaker interaction evaluative theory of stuttering (Johnson, 1967; Johnson et al., 1959) is pertinent to the investigation of the parents' attitude. In Johnson's discussion, the data of Davis (1939) and of others (Branscom, Hughes, & Oxtoby, 1955; Egland, 1955) indicating that all children are disfluent (those studied showed a wide range of variation) are cited to show that, statistically speaking, disfluency is normal. During and following the time when these studies of disfluency in the speech of children were being done, three major studies of the onset and development of stuttering were conducted (Darley, 1955; Johnson et al., 1942; Johnson et al., 1959) at the University of

More Usual

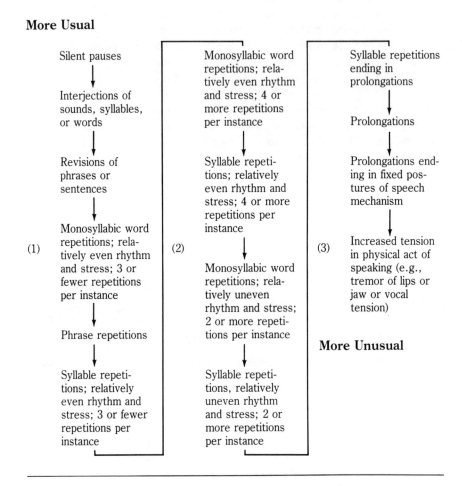

Figure 1.   Continuum of disfluent speech behaviors.

Iowa. These investigations confirmed the importance of parent-listener reactions in the origin of stuttering and showed how other attitudes in parents, particularly in mothers, might cluster with sensitive attitudes about speech.

In all these investigations, a total of 246 children judged by their parents to be stutterers, and their parents (the experimental group), along with an equal number of children judged by their parents to be nonstutterers, and their parents (the control group), were studied. Research data were compiled from

(1) Typical disfluencies that occur in preschool children's speech. Listed on the continuum in general order of expected frequency (i.e., silent pauses are the most frequent).

(2) Borderline atypical disfluencies that occur less frequently in the speech of children. In a speech sample of 500 words or more, if there are 2 or more of any one of these behaviors per 100 words, this should be considered a basis for concern, especially if air flow or phonation is disrupted between the repetitions or if a schwa-sounding vowel is substituted for the one ordinarily used in the repetition of a syllable (e.g., "Məməməmama"). May be referred to as "cross-over behaviors" on the continuum between "more usual" and "more unusual" speech disfluencies.

(3) Atypical disfluencies that are very infrequent in the speech of children. More characteristic of what listeners perceive as stuttering. If 1 or more prolongations occur per 100 words in a speech sample of 500 words or more, this should be considered a basis for considerable concern. Of course, fixed postures or other signs of increased tension and fragmentation of the flow of speech should be given immediate attention.

From Gregory and Hill (1980, p. 354). Copyright 1980 by H. Gregory and D. Hill. Reprinted by permission.

Figure 1.   Continued.

carefully planned interviews, clinical observations, and test procedures. Children in the experimental group were seen, on the average, 2½ years after the perceived onset of stuttering. Johnson realized the limitations of this research procedure since it relies on the memory of parents and the ability of an interviewer and interviewee to communicate accurately. As Bloodstein (1969) has said, "His defense of the method was in essence: If you don't study it this way, how do you study it?" (p. 221). In general, 85% to 90% of the parents agreed that the speech behavior originally diagnosed as stuttering was the effortless, brief repetition of syllables, whole words, or phrases.

The studies of normal fluency development and the onset of stuttering led Johnson to propose and advocate that stuttering was a diagnostic problem (i.e., it was not a problem until after a listener evaluated normal disfluency as stuttering and began to react to it). A second step in the process of normally disfluent speech becoming a problem was the internalization of the parents' evaluation by the child. Significantly, Johnson et al. (1959) pointed out that parents were not to blame: they were only reflecting a cultural attitude toward the fluency of speech. Furthermore, the reason that stuttering tended to run in families was that a particular sensitivity about disfluency was present in the families of stutterers (Bloodstein, Jaeger, & Tureen, 1952). In addition to the previously cited finding that the parents of stuttering children had more demanding expectations with regard to the fluency of their children, the onset studies and related studies of parental attitude (Darley, 1955; Johnson et al., 1959) appeared to show that the stuttering group's parents, especially the mothers, were more perfectionistic, more striving, and less satisfied with themselves and their children than parents of nonstutterers. These latter findings, Johnson reasoned, along with similar reports on the parents of stuttering children by Glasner (1949) and Moncur (1952), added to a picture of sensitive, hyperreactive parents.

In the last of the three onset and development studies (Johnson et al., 1959), findings relative to type of disfluency showed that sound or syllable repetitions, prolongations of sounds, word repetitions, phrase repetitions, and broken words occurred significantly more often in stuttering children, whereas stuttering and nonstuttering children had about the same number of revisions, incomplete phrases, and interjections such as "well" and "and uh." These results, and findings from listener reaction studies that sound and syllable repetitions and prolongations are more likely to be labeled as stuttering, seem to have influenced Johnson et al. (1959) to hypothesize in some of his last writing that stuttering was the result of a general interaction between three major variables: (1) the listener's sensitivity to the child's disfluency, (2) the child's degree of disfluency, and (3) the child's sensitivity to his or her own disfluency and sensitivity to the listener's evaluations. Johnson's extensive work will be cited again later, but it has been reviewed here as a rationale for obtaining a clear statement of the problem as it is perceived by parents.

Family History of Stuttering

For many years, we have been aware, based on case history information and the results of many studies, that the incidence of stuttering is significantly higher in the families of stutterers than in the families of nonstutterers (Bloodstein 1981; Sheehan & Costley, 1977; Van Riper, 1982). Twenty-five years ago there was a strong belief that this could be due to environmental influences (i.e., a concern and sensitivity about stuttering running in families). While this is still a possibility, and one to be dealt with in the prevention of stuttering, progress in the development of genetic models and research has led to increased acceptance of the idea that a genetic factor may function to predispose some children to stuttering (Kidd, 1983). Investigators such as Andrews and Harris (1964), Howie (1981), and Kidd (1980), who have reported evidence of genetic factors, assume that environmental factors interact with genetic predispositions. We are still left, as Bloodstein (1975) says, with the difficult question of what is inherited and how this can relate to intervention. Gregory (1979b) stated that the motolinguistic conditions that have been hypothesized to be related to stuttering may be a reflection of a genetic basis. In a very recent analysis, Kidd (1983) states that for some individuals a primary problem of unknown etiology may exist and that stuttering, delay in talking, and articulation difficulties are only different manifestations of this underlying problem.

It is important to find out about the family history of stuttering for what this may tell us about the likelihood of a parental sensitivity about disfluency or the possibility of a genetic link, especially as the latter may be associated with a syndrome of stuttering and language disorders. With reference to a child's regaining of normal fluency, either without formal therapy or with appropriate treatment, some speech-language pathologists believe the prognosis may be better when there is no genetic predisposition. On the other hand, we have seen families in which the parents accepted the "family tendency" and the "problem," they interacted appropriately with the child, and the child developed normally fluent speech quite readily.

General Development and Medical Factors

Information about the child's general developmental history and conditions requiring medical attention is important to obtain because delayed physical development and motor coordination or illness may be associated with delayed speech and language development or impaired motor control of the speech mechanism, which could contribute to disrupted fluency. Group studies, such as the onset studies by Johnson et al. (1959) and the more recent one by Andrews and Harris (1964), which focused on birth conditions, diseases, and early physical development, have shown that there is little in the case history of the typical stutterer that could be considered unusual. However, following an extensive critical analysis of case history studies, Bloodstein (1969) concluded that there is some evidence of more abnormal birth conditions and allergies in stutterers. He said this was ". . . interesting in the light of the relationship they [these conditions] may have to such traits as anxiety, restlessness, and emotional lability in children" (p. 176). Diagnostic experience indicates that remarkable findings in one area of the history are more or less meaningful depending on findings in related categories of the history and evaluation. Thus, significant factors may be found in this part of an individual child's history even though group comparison of physical developmental and health factors in stutterers and nonstutterers has been essentially inconclusive.

Speech and Language Development

As Van Riper points out, "It is a long step from the single-word utterances of the one-year-old to the multiple-word phrases and sentences of adult speech" (1963, p. 319). A central thesis of this study is that fluency, like articulation, is a developmental dimension of speech and that certain factors can be hazards to fluency. A delay in the development of language or articulation, combined perhaps with communicative stress or drive to express oneself, can bring about greater disfluency. We have observed that children who have had expressive language problems go through periods of increased disfluency as the condition improves. Recent reports (Hall, 1977; Merits-Patterson & Reed, 1981) have offered additional evidence of this pattern.

An early investigation of the developmental histories of stuttering children by Berry (1938) indicated that stutterers were retarded in the development of speech. In discussing stutterers' profiles, Berry and Eisenson (1956) observed that the histories of many stutterers reveal retarded onset of speech and delayed maturation of articulation. Bloodstein (1958) reported that approximately one third of 108 stuttering children examined in a cross-sectional study were described by their parents as "late talkers" or as having indistinct speech before they began to stutter. In this regard, Johnson et al. (1959) made an interesting observation in reporting on the last of the three onset studies. He stated that ". . . more experimental than control group children were rated by their mothers as 'much slower than average' in acquiring speech, but . . . there were no corresponding group differences reflected in the mean ages, reported by the mothers, at which the first words and sentences were spoken" (Johnson et al., 1959, p. 224). Johnson thought this reflected a tendency by the stutterers' parents to rate their children somewhat less favorably than objective data appeared to warrant. Andrews and Harris (1964), in a longitudinal study of 43 stuttering children and a cross-sectional comparison of 80 stuttering children and 80 controls in England, reported that stutterers were significantly late in talking. Furthermore, the stutterers were found to have a much higher incidence of developmental articulatory problems. Andrews and Harris pointed out that their population represented a cross section of an industrial city, whereas the Iowa population of Johnson's studies was from a higher socioeconomic level. They thought this difference could account for the difference in findings cited. More recently Pratt (1972) evaluated the articulatory and language skills of 17 stutterers between the ages of 3 and 5 and matched controls. She found that stutterers scored significantly lower on the Templin-Darley Screening Test of Articulation and the Peabody Picture Vocabulary Test (expressive language). The nonstutterers formulated significantly more sentences with multiple clauses. Lastly, a survey of clinicians reported by Blood and Seider (1981) has indicated that children who stutter tend to have a higher incidence of problems of articulation and language.

With reference to differential evaluation, there is much to think about here and to investigate more thoroughly. It seems evident that delayed language and speech development alone or combined with other factors may occasion an unusual degree or quality of disfluency in some children. Furthermore, information in this segment of the history takes on special meaning if the clinical evaluation reveals that the child has a language problem.

In addition, as the milestones of speech and language development are assessed, the interviewer can obtain information about the course of fluency development. Depending on the child's age, I ask about disfluency during the period when children begin to combine words (18 to 24 months), the periods when vocabulary and syntax are developing rapidly (24 to 30 months and 30 to 36 months), and the latter period and beyond when the practical use of speech is increasing. Parents or other informants may find it helpful, in giving history information, for the clinician to explain the diagram of disfluencies in Figure 1 and to model single-syllable word repetition, part-word syllable repetition, prolongation, etc. In this regard, Van Riper's description of tracks of development provides the clinician with useful frames of reference for thinking about the nature of disfluency at the designated time of the onset of stuttering and during the developmental course of stuttering (Van Riper, 1982). It is well to remember that fluency is ordinarily quite unstable during this period of rapid speech development. Increases in disfluency may be cyclical, and the clinician should note any change toward longer or shorter periods of increased disfluency, the latter obviously being a positive development.

Environmental Conditions

Although most theorists, regardless of specific points of view, have considered environmental influences important in the development of stuttering, it was Johnson who stressed that the crucial difference between a child who becomes a stutterer and one who does not is found in the parents' and others' reactions.

Others, such as Sheehan (1958a, 1968) and Glasner (1970), in tracing the beginning of stuttering and in showing how the behavior is perpetuated, have stressed the child's general feelings about himself or herself in relating to the environment. Sheehan believes that repetitions and prolongations in speech represent approach-avoidance conflict (Dollard & Miller, 1950; Miller 1944), which can have its origin in one of five levels and, in addition, can be generalized from one of these levels to another. These levels of conflict are: (1) ego protective (i.e., how the child feels about himself or herself); (2) relationship (i.e., acceptance or rejection of certain interpersonal relationships); (3) emotional loading of speech (expressing or inhibiting feelings); (4) situation-speech conflict; and (5) word-level conflict. Disfluent or stuttering behaviors are increased if conflicts are not reduced. Moreover, fear and conflict reduction that occurs simultaneously with and immediately following stuttering reinforces the behavior. Thus, approach-avoidance behavior causes stuttering; and fear reduction, at the moment the stuttering occurs, reinforces it. In this connection, Wischner (1950), in relating Johnson's diagnosogenic theory to learning theory concepts, referred to the way in which behavior, designed to avoid noxious environmental reactions to disfluency, was reinforced by momentary anxiety reduction.

Wyatt's (1969) multidisciplinary approach to the study of individual children who developed stuttering has led to her interpretation of stuttering as a loss of parental love, corrective feedback, or modeling of appropriate language forms during the development of language through the presymbolic (babbling), symbolic (naming, words), and relational (phrases, sentences) stages. The loss of feedback, causing compulsive repetition of initial sounds and syllables (which is least characteristic of normal development), is most detrimental when the child is moving from one stage of language development to the next.

Skinner's behavioral principles (Skinner, 1953) have been stressed by Shames and Sherrick (1963) in postulating that effects of the environment produce stuttering. Disfluency and stuttering are considered operant responses that are similar and continuous. Disfluency results from, among other things, maturational factors and the stress that the child experiences in communication. Aversive stimuli from a listener, which, if response-contingent, would be expected to reduce disfluency, do not, since social reactions are not that precise. In addition, the listener, the situation, and other aspects of the stimulus complex present become aversive through association and thus evoke more disfluency. The continuation of this process degenerates the speech response into what we call stuttering. Stuttering responses followed by positive reinforcers are increased. Parental, social, negative, and positive reinforcers are presented on a complex schedule, thus explaining what every clinician knows who tries to analyze the reinforcing factors that operate in a stuttering child's environment.

Brutten and Shoemaker's (1967) theoretical explanation of stuttering, which notes individual differences in autonomic reactivity and conditionability, also emphasizes the role of the environment. Their concept is that fluency, the predominant characteristic of normal speech, is disrupted by learned, classically conditioned emotionality, which increases fluency failures (repetitions and prolongations). Unadaptive instrumental or behavioral or operant responses that reduce emotional responses are reinforced, adding to the complexity of failure in fluency.

Studies of the incidence of stuttering in different cultures and socioeconomic groups have additional implications for our evaluation of environmental factors. Surveys of Indian tribes in America and other societies (Lemert, 1953, 1962; Snidecor, 1947; Stewart, 1960) have provided strong evidence that there is more stuttering in competitive, status-conscious societies in which higher standards of behavior are the rule. For example, Lemert (1962) inferred that the low incidence of stuttering in Polynesian societies and the comparatively high incidence in Japan were due to the differences in pressures to achieve and conform. Morgenstern (1956) concluded that socioeconomic upward mobility was pressure that increased stuttering in some occupational classes.

Elsewhere I have described the significance of environmental events with reference to communicative stress and interpersonal stress (Gregory, 1973b, 1984; Gregory & Hill, 1980, 1984). Communicative stress refers to the way in which the parents or others talk to the child, and interpersonal stress refers to the general interaction among family members. Case studies show that either of these two kinds of stress can increase disfluency and stuttering; and as the literature review has revealed, many writers have emphasized that one or both of these factors should be considered in the description of the problem and the case history. Specifically, we are interested in what conditions disturb speech and what conditions relax speech. Does just "Father" or "Father getting angry" occasion more disfluency or stuttering? Does playing with the child in a quiet, unhurried manner increase the child's fluency? Does talking more slowly to the child have a positive effect? Are there environmental conditions that reinforce stuttering responses (e.g., when the child finally gets the parents' attention as he or she stutters in some situation)? Are such things as parental disagreement, sibling rivalry, or discipline practices causing conflict that affects the stuttering? Are the parents in disagreement about certain aspects of the "speech problem"? Do the parents feel an unusual degree of guilt about their child-rearing practices or their reactions to the child's speech?

A parent may have too high a level of expectation related to speech development or to behavior in general, such as table manners. The parents may be demanding too much and providing too little support, which Sheehan (1970, 1975) has called an unfavorable demand/support ratio. Other factors, such as hectic or inconsistent family routine, can be discovered in the case history and related to direct observation of the child and parents.

Educational Progress

Information about the school-age child's academic progress or learning deficits may provide leads to factors that either contributed to the onset of the stuttering or, more importantly, are indirectly operating to maintain stuttering by adding to the child's present frustration. My observations agree with Bloodstein's (1958) that the beginning of stuttering in a noteworthy number of cases accompanies the child's learning to read and other confrontations with the world of language tools.

Schindler (1955) found in a small sample of stutterers in elementary school that oral reading skills were retarded by approximately 1 year. Bloodstein's review (1969) indicated that only one of five studies of the silent reading ability of stutterers had found them retarded compared to nonstutterers.

Parents also report that the social situation of the school aggravates a previously noted fluency difference. Of course, environmental conditions in the school that occasion more or less stuttering need to be studied just as they are in the home situation.

Formal Observation and Testing

Included in formal observation and testing are observation of the subject's attitude, an analysis of speech fluency, an analysis of parent-child interaction, evaluation of articulation and language, and motor testing.

Subject's Attitude

In defining stuttering, most clinical observers and researchers agree that the speaker's attitude or feeling about speech is one of the critical factors in stuttering. After obtaining information from the parents about their perception of the child's speech behavior and the way in which they believe the child is reacting, the examiner makes his or her own observations. Pertinent observations of the child's enjoyment of talking can be made throughout the evaluation, but some discussion of talking has been found to be acceptable and valuable. Williams (1969) has reported that all children have attitudes toward talking that they can express in reply to such questions as: How do you like talking? What do you like most (least) about talking? In what situations do you like to talk most (least)? I have found that talking with the child about talking, and not talking about stuttering or speech problems, is very valuable. When this approach is used, some children with obvious struggle behavior will report very little that can be considered a negative attitude toward social interaction through speech.

Video and audio tape recordings of speaking and, if appropriate, of reading should be made in circumstances that can be duplicated later for comparison. Since there are situational differences in the occurrence of disfluency and stuttering, recordings are made routinely in such situations as monologue, dialogue, play, and play with pressure. If a child is reported to show increased disfluency in a particular situation (e.g., when eating with the family), then the clinician should arrange to get an audio recording. The parent-child interaction analysis, described in the next section, may also be used as a speech sample.

The following are brief descriptions of situations used to sample speech:

Monologue. The clinician encourages the child to talk about a favorite game or television program. With some children, the clinician and the child look at pictures; then the child, following the clinician's model, describes the activity depicted in the pictures.

Dialogue. The clinician encourages the child to share interests or experiences as they talk together. The clinician may model, for example, by saying, "I have a bicycle and I like to ride. Do you have a bike?" Topics range from favorite toys or television programs to friends and family members.

Play. The clinician engages the child in a play situation on the floor. A toy village (with stores, cars, people) or a dollhouse are used.

Play with pressure. The clinician continues to engage the child in play but now systematically interjects verbal interference for about 5 minutes—by either increasing speech rate, interrupting and challenging, loosing eye contact, hurrying the child, or misunderstanding the child. Obviously, these pressures are not done all at once.

Tapes are analyzed noting the type and number of disfluencies, including those defined as stuttering. Our goal is to obtain a sample of at least 500 words, but the disfluencies are recorded in terms of type per 100 words. For use in clinical evaluation, I use the continuum of disfluent speech behaviors from *More Usual* to *More Unusual* (see Figure 1) as a guide in making a judgment about a child's speech and in determining the degree of concern. This continuum is based on quantitative and qualitative information available about disfluency and stuttering (reviewed in an earlier section), my clinical experience, and the clinical experience of others such as Cooper (1973), Van Riper (1982), and Yairi (1981). I like the continuum idea because it reflects our present knowledge about children's disfluency and because the use of "concern" in describing evaluation lends itself to a consideration of degree (Gregory, 1984a, 1984b). Our judgment about the child's speech—typical, borderline atypical, or atypical—is, as we will see, an important consideration in prescribing therapy.

Some stutterer's speech is characterized not only by the disfluency types mentioned above and their accessory behaviors but also by a rapid, slurred, and jerky pattern often typified by the running together of words. This behavior has been termed *cluttering* and is referred to by some clinicians as "poorly organized speech" because of the impression one gets when listening. Clinicians and researchers with a European background (Freund, 1966; Weiss, 1964) have described this type of fluency-articulation pattern in greater detail, but we American-trained speech-language pathologists, becoming more interested in the problem, are beginning to report seeing it clinically. Of course, there may be cluttering without stuttering or with only minimal stuttering. Since this speech behavior is often described as associated with a language problem, it will be discussed more thoroughly in the next section.

The clinician may also evaluate the child's response to the clinician's modeling of what we call "easy relaxed approach with smooth movement" on words and phrases using a direct model (i.e., the clinician says "ball," the child says "ball"). The initial consonant-vowel or vowel-consonant combination in a word or the first word of a phrase is produced with a relaxed, smooth movement that is slightly slower than usual. To increase the child's attention, I may say, "Watch me. Can you tell your speech to do this?" This procedure reflects the finding that disfluency or stuttering is more likely to occur at the beginning of a word or a clause. At this point, we are merely observing the child's ability to attend to and follow a model.

Parent-Child Interaction Analysis

In taking the case history we collect information about psychosocial factors that may be important. As we saw in discussing the rationale for investigating environmental influences, there is considerable clinical and research information to indicate that more specific procedures are needed. Parent-child interaction evaluation procedures, first explored by Kasprisin (1970), Kasprisin-Burrelli, Egolf, and Shames (1972), and more recently Mordecai (1979), appear to be a promising way to add to or confirm case history reports. Clinicians learn to reliably identify the parent's positive and negative child-directed behaviors. Although it is ideal to analyze videotaped samples of recorded nonverbal reactions precisely, an audiotaped sample of verbal interaction is adequate.

The parent-child interaction is partially structured by such activities as playing with a toy village or a dollhouse, putting together a puzzle, or playing an appropriate game such as lotto. The following parental behaviors are examples of those that are probably significant in developing and maintaining of stuttering: interruption, asking many questions, asking a second question before the initial one has been answered, asked multiple questions, filling in words, finishing a child's statement, guessing what the child is about to say, constant correction of the child's verbal and nonverbal behavior, and speech models of rapidly paced conversation that includes quick changes in topics. These behaviors are counted, and a profile of positive and negative behaviors are used by the clinician as a frame of reference in modeling suggested modifications for the parents.

Evaluation of Articulation and Language

Articulation, the production of speech sounds, should be tested by following procedures that vary depending on the age of the subject (Schwartz, 1983). Evaluating connected speech, as well as single words in isolation, gives the examiner the opportunity to listen for the consistency of articulation errors and disfluencies or to perceive any cluttering present. The rationale for this testing has been established by the previously reported finding that meaningful numbers of stuttering children have articulation problems (Andrews & Harris, 1964) or are reported by their parents to have had indistinct speech before they began to stutter (Bloodstein, 1958). When an articulation problem exists with disfluency or stuttering, speech pathologists frequently ask which they should work with first. As we will see later in this section and the one on therapy, the correct question is perhaps this: what is the correct way to work with both of these?

A related aspect of the formal clinical evaluation is an assessment of receptive and expressive language. As stated earlier, it appears probable that delayed oral language development can be associated with the occurrence of an unusual degree or quality of disfluency in some children. Moreover, difficulty with reading may become associated with difficulty in speaking and lead to more disfluency (or increased stuttering) during the early school years. Bloodstein (1958, 1969) has also emphasized these conditions in his description of stuttering as an anticipatory struggle reaction. According to Bloodstein, stuttering begins as a response of tension and fragmentation of speech, not greatly different from certain other disfluencies. This happens under various circumstances in which the child comes to have the conviction that speech demands unusual precaution. He states: "On the basis of clinical evidence it appears possible that retarded language development, articulation errors, reading difficulty, cluttering, difficulties of phonation, or practically any other kind of verbal ineptness or obstacle to communication may render a child more or less chronically subject to the threat of speech failure . . ." (1969, p. 44). Bloodstein adds that it is more likely that these factors will take effect if the child is subjected to excessive parental demands for more adequate speech or if the child has a tendency to be sensitive or fearful. Luper (1968) has also linked the stability of a child's language skills, among other factors, to the child's tolerance threshold for withstanding excess tension of the speech musculature. This point of view coincides with my own: that some children with varying degrees of a stuttering problem may have word-finding or syntactic problems that should be accounted for in a careful differential evaluation (Gregory, 1973, 1984a, 1984b; Gregory & Hill, 1980). Furthermore, Bloodstein's theory postulates, as does the thesis of this monograph, that factors that may be the beginning of stuttering are to a degree the same factors that cause disfluency in all children.

Disfluency is a feature of expressive oral language. However, since expression presupposes reception and, to a great extent, organizational mediating processes, these functions are evaluated also. Among tests that have been used for this purpose are the Peabody Picture Vocabulary Test (Dunn, 1965), the Illinois Test of Psycholinguistic Ability (Kirk, McCarthy, & Kirk, 1968), the Northwestern Syntax Screening Test (Lee, 1969), and the Carrow Test of Auditory Comprehension for Language and the Carrow Elicited Language Inventory (Carrow, 1974).

While focusing on a discussion of language, we should give additional consideration to cluttering, which has been related to language dysfunction. The literature on the subject contains much conjecture based on clinical observation, but very little research has focused on the etiology, description, and development of cluttering. However, there appears to be agreement that the rapid, slurred, jerky, indistinct pattern characteristic of cluttering is related to a general language disability. Freund (1966) stresses an imbalance between the drive to communicate and the child's ability. Apparently if need and potential were more in balance, speech would be better. In this way, cluttering may also be related to environmental factors. Arnold (1965) concludes that cluttering is an inherited, organically determined language problem associated with a lack of musical ability, diminished discriminatory and interpretative ability in the auditory modality, delayed motoric development, and possibly deficient lateral dominance. Weiss (1964) has postulated that stuttering develops as an attempt on the part of a child to avoid cluttering. Some years ago he observed that when stuttering is relieved, a cluttering-like residue remains. In working with children, and more clearly with adults, I have found the cluttering element present in problems of stuttering. Children with stuttering-cluttering behavior are often those who show articulation and language problems of mild to moderate degrees.

Central auditory processing is a function that is thought to be related to language facility and the motor patterning of speech. In addition, since delayed auditory feedback disrupts speech production including fluency, there has been a historical interest in auditory functioning as related to stuttering (Gregory & Mangan, 1982). Although there are some contradictory research findings, adult stutterers show signs of minimal auditory processing problems based on the use of such procedures as dichotic listening employing meaningful linguistic stimuli (Curry & Gregory, 1969; Quinn, 1972; Sommers, Brady, & Moore, 1975), auditory test batteries (Hall & Jerger, 1978; Toscher & Rupp, 1978), and auditory-motor tracking (Sussman & MacNeilage, 1975). (Regarding dichotic listening, Kimura [1967] has shown that when verbal symbols such as digits or words are heard simultaneously in both ears, or dichotically, most subjects are more successful at reporting words heard at the right ear than at the left.) One hypothesis is that we are detecting a minimal problem of auditory memory and feedback that is related to the child's ability to recall auditorily and to hold sequences of sounds in mind until a series is completed. In this regard, our interest is perhaps closely related to that of Wingate. He finds in a series of studies (Wingate, 1966, 1967, 1971) evidence that a substantial number of adult stutterers show deficits in the skill of manipulating sounds or sound patterns. Earlier, Stromsta (1959) and Tormatis (1956) offered research results that they believed indicate that a disturbance in auditory feedback processes disrupts the integrated forward flow of speech in some stutterers. Obviously the auditory system of children needs to be studied. With patience and care auditory-evoked responses can be used with children, and since this procedure does not involve a behavioral response, it may be used to provide more information about the auditory system and stuttering (see Decker, Healey, & Howe, 1982).

Motor Testing

Some clinical cases in which stuttering, or possible stuttering, is the focal point in our evaluation have been found to have minimal problems of motor control or patterning for the production of speech. Riley and Riley (1983) report that 61% of a public school sample of children who stutter had an observable oral-motor discoordination. Our clinical sample reveals a somewhat lesser number, 25%. Testing procedures and criteria used may account in part for the variation in findings. Diadochokinetic rates, the sequential chaining of syllables such as "puhtuhkuh," and a careful oral examination are used to determine the importance of this factor in individual cases. Nonspeech gross motor skills are observed using selected tasks from Gesell and Armatruda (1948) and such instruments on the Osretsky Test of Motor Proficiency (Doll, 1947a). These findings are compared to those on general development and the development of speech and language from the case history and the more formal evaluation of articulation and language.

This topic cannot be left without discussing briefly the tremendous interest during recent years of the possible contribution of minimal motor factors on the development of stuttering. In reaction time studies employing brief verbal responses (vowels or consonant-vowel combinations), the general conclusion is that stutterers show longer latencies (Starkweather, 1982). Some evidence for a more general or overall minimal motor difference is Luper and Cross's (1978) finding that stutterers (5-year-olds, 9-year-olds, and adults) differ from matched nonstutterers on both a voice reaction time task and a finger reaction time response. The correlations of scores on the two types of tasks were very high: +.96 for the stutterers and +.88 for the nonstutterers. It should be noted that Reich, Till, and Goldsmith (1981), in a study similar to that of Luper and Cross that used adult subjects only, found a difference between stutterers and non-stutterers on speech reaction time, but not for forefinger button-pressing or a throat-clearing cough. They concluded that the longer speech reaction times exhibited by the stutterers "reflect learned anticipatory fears of phonatory initiation and maladaptive prephonatory muscular sets" (p. 195). In other words, emotional conditioning could be involved in the minimal motor reaction time differences found. The problem of separating out these factors (i.e., determining whether a motor response difference is due to neurophysiological factors or minimal emotional factors) seems to be a very formidable one.

There are two problems involved in gathering meaningful research to clarify information about motor functioning related to stuttering: (1) minimal differences in stutterers are difficult to establish because there is so much overlap with test data on nonstutterers, and (2) it is difficult to use research instruments to study the speech production of children. Conture's (1984) research exemplifies these two difficulties. Examining spectograms, he reports a greater proportion of multiple-stop plosive release bursts on voiceless consonants in young stutterers' speech than that of matched nonstuttering children. He also observed, using electroglottography, that stuttering children showed more glottal adduction per glottic cycle, compared again to match nonstuttering children. However, nonstuttering control subjects showed enough of both of these characteristics to make one skeptical about the clinical significance of this difference. Conture speculates that youngsters who stutter are at the lower end of the continuum of normally proficient talkers in terms of motor efficiency for speech production.

Related Examination Procedures

The examination procedures that have been discussed are clearly within the province of the speech and language pathologist. The differential evaluation of stuttering or possible stuttering problems involves other testing and observation and a close working relationship with other specialists. Much more needs to be done in fostering a multidisciplinary approach (Blaesing, 1982; Gregory, 1980).

Most children's progress is followed by a medical specialist to whom we can refer requests for information about health and development. Gaining a knowledge of environmental factors, obviously important, can be accomplished with the assistance of a social worker or school counselor. Reviews and commentaries on the literature (Goodstein, 1958; Johnson, 1967; Sheehan, 1958b), while not reporting the finding of a particular personality pattern that is characteristic of stutterers, do conclude that stutterers appear somewhat more anxious, tense, and withdrawn. Moreover, psychosocial factors have been stressed by most clinicians and researchers in one way or another as being important in the development of stuttering. Consequently, the psychologist's use of techniques such as the Children's Apperception Test (Bellak, 1954) is likely to help in understanding more subtle attitudes in stuttering children that we may not perceive. More information on perceptual and intellectual functioning that will relate to our study of speech and language processes can be derived from use of such procedures as the Bender Visual-Motor Gestalt Test (Bender, 1946). The Vineland Social Maturity Scale (Doll, 1947b) is useful in providing pertinent data on the development of social competence, which can be compared with or used to clarify information from the history. These are only examples of formal approaches that the psychologist can employ. In addition, it should be understood that the psychiatrist and psychologist have had experience in their work with children and parents that enables them to recognize important patterns of interaction and behavior that speech pathologists will not be so likely to see.

Early interest in neurophysiological factors in stuttering reached a high point with Travis's cerebral dominance theory (Travis, 1931) and Eisenson's explanation of stuttering as a manifestation of perseveration in speaking (Eisenson & Winslow, 1938). Travis (1957) moved to a more psychodynamic conception of stuttering, but he has been very interested in the previously discussed findings of dichotic listening differences in stutterers as these results may reflect less lateral brain dominance in stutterers.

Regarding electroencephalographic research, Luchsinger and Landolt (1951) reported that clutterers and clutterer-stutterers had slightly pathological EEGs. Fox (1966) and Graham (1966) found adult stutterers to have normal brain waves. Recently the development of better technology including computer analysis of data has resulted in new approaches and new observations. For example, Moore and Haynes (1980) and Moore and Lorendo (1980) have reported that stutterers as a group show more suppression of alpha activity over the right hemisphere immediately preceding an overt language task or when listening to speech; in contrast, nonstuttering control subjects show more suppression over the left hemisphere as expected in terms of cerebral dominance for language. These findings are often related to the finding of dichotic listening differences between stutterers and nonstutterers in which stutterers show smaller between-ear differences and more reversals (i.e., better left-ear scores) when meaningful linguistic stimuli are used (Gregory & Mangan, 1982). There may be meaning in those findings as related to our interest in genetic factors (Kidd, 1980) and observations of more language delay and articulation problems in children who stutter.

Presently it is concluded that routine clinical neurological examination does not appear warranted. However, in the speech and language evaluation and in the psychological evaluation when they are part of a multidisciplinary evaluation, these EEG findings related to language processing mean that we should look carefully at subject variables that reflect cognitive, perceptual, and motolinguistic functioning.

PART TWO

Differential Stuttering Therapy

Differential evaluation results in decisions about therapy. We have seen that information related to many aspects of the individual and his or her environment is pertinent to the making of these decisions. The onset and development of stuttering is complex, and treatment must not be fragmented. In practice, clinicians consider the information they obtain in the evaluation and decide upon a tentative course of action, which varies somewhat in every case depending on case history findings, observations, and testing. As I see it, clinicians are invited to enter into the ongoing process of events in a child's life. They hope that by joining the child, the parents, and others, the direction of the developing process toward stuttering or more serious stuttering can be changed. The initial evaluation is just the beginning of an important and perhaps rather long involvement that will produce new information, causing the clinician to modify earlier opinions.

Although the reviewed clinical observations and research findings indicate that approaches to therapy have to be modified with every case, the general areas of therapy will be discussed in terms of two differentiating factors: the developmental stage of stuttering and the person's chronological age. The prevention of stuttering and the management of early stages, mainly with regard to preschool children, will be discussed first. We shall then consider work with more confirmed stutterers approximately 10 years old or older as well as adult stutterers. Finally, the way in which these procedures are modified in working with younger stutterers of elementary school age will be considered.

Prevention and Management of Stuttering in the Early Stages

Three developments that have come out of the rapid expansion of research, training, and service activities in speech and language pathology have helped in a major way to prevent stuttering. First, parents have become better informed about speech and language development and the physical, psychological, and social factors involved. Second, parents and the public in general have gained access to information about the factors that contribute to increased disfluency and the development of stuttering. Third, speech-language pathologists have become competent in counseling parents and working with children when there is concern that children are beginning to stutter.

In certain localities where speech-language pathology is a highly developed profession (e.g., the north-shore suburbs of Chicago), there is a noticeably lower case load of children who stutter in public school programs. A major contribution has been made by the Speech Foundation of America, a nonprofit organization that has disseminated information about stuttering, including booklets on its prevention.

Gregory (1984b) has concluded that clinicians are working with the following factors in their attempts to prevent the development of stuttering or, as we say in talking to parents, "stemming the tide of development during early stages":

1. Communicative stress in the environment (i.e., the way in which the parents and other adults talk to the child and the rate of the parents' speech)
2. Interpersonal stress (i.e., the general ways in which family members interact with each other)
3. Linguistic and motor developmental differences
4. Speech fluency

We assume that the first three of these factors influence the fourth, speech fluency, but a recent development has been to give more attention to procedures that focus more specifically on speech fluency, such as the clinician modeling smoother-flowing speech for the child. The main thesis of this presentation is that different child variables (3 above) and environmental variables (1 and 2 above) will be emphasized to the extent determined by the initial evaluation and subsequent treatment.

A tentative therapy program for working with a child and the parents is determined following an evaluation. For illustrative purposes, consider the following two children:

A. Bill (48 months)

Onset: Around his third birthday, parents were concerned about stuttering that included tense repetitions of sounds and syllables.

Speech analysis: Moderately severe stuttering problem characterized by tense repetitions of sounds, syllables, and words (mostly of one syllable). Some prolongations noted and some repetitions ended in prolongations. Articulation was slightly indistinct but at age level.

Developmental factors: General physical development was normal. Described as a quiet baby. Babbled during the first year, imitated sounds of toys and gestured at 12–15 months. Spoke first words at 18–20 months. Used pointing to communicate and one- or two-word utterances until about 2 years 6 months, when sentences began to develop. Evaluation revealed receptive language was at age level, but expressive language was below age level and characterized by presentence constructions, the omission of verbs, etc. Diadokokinetic rates of tongue and lip movement were judged to be slightly below average.

Environmental factors: Bill plays well with his older brother and neighborhood children. Both parents regularly take time to play with him. He is generally happy and well behaved. Mother is trying to "maintain a more calm, relaxed atmosphere in the home." Stuttering increases when he is playing with peers or when he is excited.

B. Warren (3 years, 11 months)

Onset: About the time of his third birthday, parents and a neighborhood mother noted stuttering that consisted of the repetition of initial syllables in words. Four months later when parents returned from a trip, "Warren was stuttering all of the time."

Speech analysis: Repetitions of sounds, syllables, and one-syllable words at the beginning of a phrase. Repetitions characterized by relatively even rhythm. Occasionally, there were short breaths between repetitions. There were only a few prolongations. Stuttering classified as mild, consisting of borderline atypical disfluencies. Was able to imitate a model of easy, relaxed speech readily and some immediate carry-over was noted.

Developmental factors: All developmental milestones, including speech and language, essentially normal. No significant medical problems. Clinical evaluation revealed speech and language abilities within normal range. Psychological evaluation resulted in an IQ of 105, which the psychologist thought was probably lower than his actual operating level since several failures on tasks represented "resistance to the task and attention problems." Index of social maturity 1 year below age level. Psychologist concluded that child was over-anxious and insecure emotionally.

Environmental factors: Mother described Warren as loving, sensitive, and intelligent. She also said he was anxious, aggressive, sometimes stubborn, and "a boy who requires a great deal of discipline." Parents consulted pediatrician a few months earlier about child's temper tantrums. He is often in the care of a live-in housekeeper. Mother suspects that "he acts out to get attention." During last year he has been in nursery school where there have been no behavior problems.

In managing the stuttering of Bill, the emphasis was on facilitating language skills through the use of naming activities and, as this improved, the building of syntactic structures. Attention was given to oral-motor coordination employing drills in which syllables and words were chained together. The clinician modeled a more easy, relaxed speech pattern beginning with words and working up to longer, more meaningful utterances. Work on language was coordinated with therapy directed toward improving speech flow. The parents were counseled to understand therapy and the developmental factors contributing to Bill's stuttering as well as how these were being dealt with in therapy. The parents learned to modify their speech rate and to be relaxed in taking turns with the child during conversation. Therapy on a regular basis ended after 18 months.

In managing the stuttering of Warren, our principal concern was his emotional-social development and parent-child relationships. Parents and child were seen for therapy for a 3-month period during which the psychological evaluation (mentioned in the case description) was done. Warren responded well to the clinician's model of easy relaxed speech. The mother learned to adopt a slower, more relaxed speaking rate and was encouraged to follow the clinician's model of quietly setting behavioral limits and turn-taking in conversation. When the mother entered the therapy room to participate in activities, Warren would cling to her and become more disfluent. Based on observations in the clinic and the psychological evaluation, the child and the parents were referred for family-oriented psychotherapy, in which Warren was seen alone and the parents were seen for counseling. Following 4 months of psychotherapy the psychologist reports that he seldom notices any unusual disfluency. Warren is described as working through his fears and insecurities. He clings to his mother much less than before. The mother understands her role better and is not being manipulated by the child as much. The psychologist concludes, "He's going to be O.K." We don't expect to see Warren again at the speech clinic, but we will follow up. These two simplified examples show how differential evaluation indicates different therapeutic methods. As indicated in the next section, many of the cases we see are less complicated than these examples and require only preventive or prescriptive parent counseling over a period of 2 to 10 weeks. The remainder of this section will consider special topics related to prevention and early intervention.

Three General Treatment Strategies

Historically we have recognized that the length and intensity of therapy required for successful results varies from child to child (Cooper, 1979; Luper & Mulder, 1964; Van Riper, 1963, 1973). Gregory (1984a) and Gregory and Hill (1980, 1984) have described three treatment strategies that relate to the nature and degree of the child's disfluency or stuttering and the presence of complicating speech, language, or behavior problems. These three strategies are: Preventive Parent Counseling, Prescriptive Parent Counseling, and Comprehensive Therapy Program.

In Preventive Parent Counseling, the parents are seen for about four sessions, if it is judged that the parents are expressing concern about disfluency that seems to be within normal limits. The objective here is to more thoroughly evaluate our initial impression, to provide information to the parents, and to make sure the parents understand and are comfortable with the problem. Prescriptive Parent Counseling involves not only the parents but, on a limited basis, the child. The parents and the child are seen for four to eight sessions on a weekly basis if the child is showing what we call borderline atypical disfluencies, if the "problem" has existed for less than a year, and if there appears to be no significant complicating speech, language, or behavioral characteristics. With the Comprehensive Therapy Program the child is seen two to four times a week and the parents for two counseling sessions a week if the child is demonstrating borderline atypical disfluency or stuttering speech that has been present for a year or longer with or without complicating speech, language, or behavioral factors.

Parent Counseling

This involves a verbal interaction with the parents to modify attitudes and to suggest environmental modifications. It also gives the clinician an opportunity to model changes for the parents in communicative and more general interpersonal interactions. In brief, effective parent counseling involves the following sequential steps:

1. Establish a permissive relationship in which the parents are rewarded for expressing their thoughts about the child and their own behavior and for attempting to put into words the way they feel.
2. Provide information about speech development and how stuttering may develop. Several possibilities about the beginning of stuttering should be described, as this has been found to relieve guilt feelings the parents might have about one particular course of action, which they may feel caused the problem. The Speech Foundation of America's publication, *Counseling Stutterers*, discusses questions parents ask in counseling sessions (Fraser-Gruss, 1981).
3. Discuss environmental factors such as communicative stress (competition in talking, unresponsive listeners, parents asking multiple questions at once, interruptions, rapid speech rate of parents, etc.) and interpersonal stress (conflict situations, general conflict between family members, excessive behavioral demands for such things as neatness, etc.). Discuss the way in which these characteristics in a particular situation may interact with characteristics of the child (language deficits, immature articulation, drive to communicate, emotional insecurity, etc.) that are hazards to fluency. Give the parents positive suggestions for reducing the disruption of fluency. It is usually not adequate to merely advise parents to ignore something about which they have concern.
4. Building on approaches described by Wyatt (1969), clinicians have learned to model ways of communicating and interacting with children that help parents to modify their behavior. Wyatt gives the following example:

   > In the presence of mother and child the therapist demonstrated games of "word matching" and "mutual imitation," derived from observing effective interaction between mothers and young children and between preschool teachers and children. The mother was encouraged to spend more time each day alone with the stuttering child in an affectionate setting of bodily closeness. Mother and child were to talk with each other in simple short sentences, in an atmosphere where each one had the other's full attention. (pp. 118–119)

   We have found that parents respond positively to the clinician modeling for them, first while they watch from behind an observation mirror, then as they participate in the clinic room. Children, in most cases, respond well as they see the parents interacting in the situation and then doing at home what has been done at the clinic.

5. Talk *with*, not *at*, the parents when exploring their feelings and needs. Don't be uncomfortable about a period of silence in talking with parents. The counseling relationship needs to be an unpressured one. Adopt the attitude that it is more important to learn from the parents than to tell them how much you know. Fraser-Gruss (1981) and Gregory (1985) provide useful information about counseling parents along the lines of this brief discussion.
6. Have parents read sections on speech interaction or nonverbal communipation in *If Your Child Stutters: A Guide for Parents* (Ainsworth & Fraser-Gruss, 1977) and *Between Parent and Child* (Ginott, 1969).

More Direct Fluency-Enhancing Procedures

As said above, in addition to working with environmental and developmental factors that impact on a child's speech fluency, there has been a trend during the last 10 years toward the use of more specific fluency-enhancing procedures. Gerory (1973a), Gregory and Hill (1980, 1984), Nelson (1984), Perkins (1979), Shine (1984), and Van Riper (1973) describe the modeling by the clinician of modifications of speech that result in normal fluency, focusing on a minimal number of parameters. At Northwestern, we model what we call easy speech, a slightly slower than normal rate with easy initiations and smooth transitions beginning with one-word responses and working up to connected speech. The model is faded gradually as the child's speech becomes more normally fluent.

Desensitization, as first described by Van Riper and Egland (Van Riper, 1963), may be used as the child's fluency becomes more stable. During a session, the child is allowed to feel this fluency; then, based on a knowledge of what appears to disrupt the child's speech, the clinician introduces fluency disruptors such as hurrying the child, interrupting, or not paying attention. The clinician works back and forth from providing a more calm, relaxed speaking situation to some degree of disruption. This procedure increases the tolerance of factors that once disrupted fluency. This is not done by the parents, only by the clinician.

Management of Complicating Speech, Language, and Behavior Factors

Procedures to facilitate fluency are usually carried out in the context of a language activity program, working from shorter to longer utterances and from less meaningful to more meaningful content. Therefore, language therapy aimed toward syntactic development or the development of vocabulary can be integrated with procedures to facilitate fluency. In addition, as a child is responding positively and fluency is improving, articulation can be focused upon using a relaxed, developmental approach.

If a child is somewhat shy and withdrawn, or aggressive, or has perfectionistic tendencies, the clinician has to respond to this behavior as well as to the child's speech and language. Children do not come in neat packages. With the shy child who does not seem to be enjoying speech, fluency is not the first concern. The clinician focuses early in therapy on creating an atmosphere in which the child enjoys speaking more. With the child who is very active and aggressive, the clinician can reward more restricted behavior after establishing rapport with the child and finding other charcteristics that can be reinforced. In the case of one child who was perfectionistic, one of our clinicians modeled making mistakes and saying, "It's O.K. to make a mistake." This approach, combined with reduced demands on the part of the parents, gave the child a more relaxed, less demanding attitude toward herself.

Therapy for Confirmed Upper School-Age or Adult Secondary Stutterers

In contrast to stuttering in the early stages of development, factors that contribute to the onset and development of stuttering are not as apparent at this stage as are acquired attitudes, learned behavior patterns, and learned secondary stuttering behaviors. As children become more aware of their stuttering, we hypothesize that some of them attempt to inhibit disfluency by tensing and controlling the speech mechanism, a behavior that most often adds to the difficulty. Speech is more of a ballistic process that is not intended to be controlled word by word or certainly not sound by sound. As tension of the vocal track increases, there is more fragmentation of speech flow until blocks occur. When the person is blocked, certain starter behaviors appear to help break the block — such as saying "Ah wa, Ah wa" (the author's most frequently used starter when he was stuttering as a young person) or jerking the head. When a sound or a word becomes the focus of difficulty, the person will substitute one word for the other. Situational avoidances develop (e.g., not making a purchase or a telephone call). Sheehan (1958a) and Wischner (1950) hypothesized that these behaviors, which accompany momentary reduction of anxiety or tension, are reinforced since anxiety-tension reduction is actually a positive reinforcer. In the technical terminology of behavior modification this is known as negative reinforcement because the response results in the removal of a punishing state (Skinner, 1953). The stutterer's fear and tension is subsequently maintained by his memory of difficulty and approach-avoidance feelings (Sheehan, 1968, 1970). Van Riper (1973) provides more details about the development of what has been designated as secondary or accessary behaviors.

In *Controversies about Stuttering Therapy* (Gregory, 1979a, 1979b) I have described the "stutter more fluently" and the "speak more fluently" models of therapy. Historically, the stutter-more-fluently approach was a reaction to procedures that enabled the stutterer to speak more fluently without coping with the perceived nature of stuttering as fear-motivated avoidance behavior. These procedures included swinging the arm in a figure eight while speaking with careful concentration on speech production, sometimes stressing one particular parameter like increased sound duration. Clinicians such as Bryngelson, Johnson, Bloodstein, Sheehan, and Van Riper (Gregory, 1979a), although differing on some details, stressed that the stutterers should not be given some method to stop stuttering and readily produce fluency, but that they should attend to their stuttering, learn to monitor the behavior, and then gradually modify the stuttering by first thinking of and seeing how they can stutter more easily. In this way, the stutterers do not avoid stuttering as much because they are studying and modifying it. Sheehan emphasized that stutterers need to perceive more realistically their dual role as a person who stutters but who also speaks normally.

During the last 20 years, replacing stuttering speech behavior with fluent speech has been studied and advocated by contributors such as Brady, Cherry and Sayers, Goldiamond, Perkins, Ryan, Webster, and Wingate (Gregory, 1979a). Various approaches such as delayed auditory feedback (DAF), the use of masking and rhythm, and the teaching of speech gestures such as rate control, easy initiation, phrasing, and blending have been used. Features of initially obtained fluency are usually modified to accomplish speech that is perceived as normal. Advocates of the stutter-more-fluently model seem to place the objective of studying and monitoring speech behavior ahead of increasing fluency in working with confirmed stutterers, whereas advocates of the speak-more-fluently model seem more interested in bringing about an efficient (rapid) increase in fluency and an efficient (rapid) decrease in stuttering. In general, they believe that the best way to reduce avoidance tendencies is for the stutterer to learn behavior that is contrary to stuttering.

During the last 20 years I have combined the two models by evolving a program of therapy (Gregory, 1968a, 1968b) in which stutterers learn first to monitor unadaptive stuttering behavior and stutter with less tension; then through relaxed speech onsets, phrasing, and so forth they learn speech skills that are counter to stuttering. A major advantage of this approach is that stutterers become less sensitive about stuttering and at the same time they begin building speech skills appropriate for normal fluency. Along the same line of combining the two approaches, Guitar and Peters (1980) give very practical suggestions for utilizing elements of stuttering modification therapy, fluency shaping therapy, or a combined approach with individual subjects. Diagnostic indications for the appropriate treatment are based on a study of the client's speech behaviors, feelings and attitudes, and trial therapy. In a recent discussion of current techniques used in England, Cheasman (1983) states that she is finding success by combining the two models in ways similar to what I have done (Gregory, 1968a, 1979a, 1979b) and to what is described by Guitar and Peters (1980).

Beginning in the 1960s (Gregory, 1968a, 1968b) I evolved a frame of reference, based mainly on learning theory concepts, for working with older secondary stutterers, age 10 to 12 and above, which includes four general areas of activity. Each area will be discussed below.

Changing the Attitudes of the Stutterer

Although the modification of overt responses can also influence attitudes, activities in this therapeutic area are focused on a clarification of thinking and learning to verbalize feelings. Early in therapy the clinician creates a permissive situation in which clients are encouraged to talk about how their problem developed, how it affects their lives now, what they have found helpful, what they believe others think about them, etc. The clinician must come across as a person who wants to understand the client's unique thoughts and feelings and who has no preconceptions about the person. As individuals begin to talk about themselves and their problem, they begin to evaluate their ideas and reorganize their thinking. It has been observed that stutterers tend to generalize from perceived punishment of stuttering to the act of discussing it. For this reason, they are reticent to talk about it, but the opportunity to talk – one of the unique aspects of therapy – helps to countercondition anxiety. Information about stuttering and the dynamics of personal adjustment helps stutterers to see new options. Finally, as their speech improves, they have to accept new challenges and responsibilities. They must understand how tendencies to rationalize certain behavior in the past, based on being people who stuttered, may obstruct conscious desires to improve (Sheehan, 1970).

Although clinicians such as Perkins (1979), who adhere more to a speak-more-fluently model, emphasize this kind of attitudinal work, advocates of the stutter-more-fluently model, or those who combine the two in various ways, are much more likely to emphasize therapeutic activity focused more specifically on attitude change. While speak-more-fluently advocates acknowledge that some stutterers have attitudinal problems that interfere with therapy, they often believe that speech change will bring about sufficient positive shifts in attitude. Bloodstein (1958), Dalton (1983), Gregory (1968a, 1968b), Sheehan (1958a, 1968, 1970), and Van Riper (1973) discuss numerous shifts in attitude that stutterers may need to make as part of the improvement process.

Diminishing Excessive Bodily Tension

Instruction in progressive and differential muscle relaxation, emphasizing the techniques of Jacobson (1938), is valuable in helping the stutterer to reduce tension during speech. In addition, the stutterer's thinking of, and striving for, relaxation when under stress seems to have the effect of bringing about a general reduction of negative emotion and excitement (Gregory, 1968a). According to Wolpe (1958), unadaptive habits such as stuttering learned in an anxiety-generating situation can be counterconditioned by responses that inhibit anxiety responses and have a calming effect. Relaxation is one response that is said to have such a reciprocally inhibiting effect. Brutten and Shoemaker (1967) and Gray and England (1969) have adapted Wolpe's reciprocal inhibition-desensitization method of psychotherapy to stuttering therapy. They use relaxation as the antagonistic response to decondition emotional responses that disorganize fluent speech. We have found relaxation work stressing an increased and differential awareness of muscular tension to be a valuable part of stuttering therapy. Specifically, as stutterers begin to modify their speech, they strive to carry more of the feeling of optimal bodily tension over into the muscles involved in speaking. When they enter a speaking situation that involves increased emotion, they think of and strive to reduce bodily tension. In many people this has a calming effect.

Analyzing and Modifying Speech

Johnson (1967) speculated that stuttering behavior confirms the secondary stutterer's expectation of difficulty. As previously noted, Sheehan (1953) and Wischner (1950) have hypothesized that the occurrence of stuttering is accompanied by a momentary reduction of general anxiety and tension. Therefore, the behavior of the stuttering block (the head jerk, eye blink, lip pressure, and the like) is reinforced. In his most recent writing, Sheehan (Sheehan & Sheehan, 1984) has once again stressed that what we see and hear a stutterer doing is an attempt to suppress stuttering.

As stutterers gain insight into the nature of stuttering and the way attitude influences their problem, increased emphasis is placed on a study of the stuttering and general pattern of speaking. A stutterer's speech is not distorted just at the more obvious moment of stuttering, but also as the stutterer approaches a "block" or following the occurrence of stuttering in segments of speech that may be considered fluent. Therefore, the speech analysis includes observations of speech rate, phrasing (including an efficient use of exhalation), and prosody, as well as specific characteristics of stuttering. Audio recordings are used at first, followed by the use of video recordings. The mirror, one of the oldest methods of all, is very useful when the person needs to identify some behavior such as eye blinking.

Identification of stuttering behaviors is followed by negative practice and gradually learning to modify stuttering by relaxing the tension, slowing the repetition, and the like. Most clients begin to experience less stuttering and more fluency during this stage of learning to stutter more easily. Next, we often stress using an easier, more relaxed approach with smooth movements, first in the initiation of words, then phrases, and then on each phrase in connected speech. Van Riper's sequence of cancellation, pull-out, and preparatory set (Van Riper, 1963, 1973) may be used. Stutterers should understand that they are counterconditioning old feelings and behaviors. When they study their stuttering, they are adopting a changed attitude of facing up to what they have tried to conceal and avoid. When voluntary disfluency is emitted (e.g., "I'm Dan Thur-Thurston"), the clinician rewards the person for using a disfluent pattern voluntarily, the type of response that the stutterer previously associated with punishment and thus feared and avoided. The rewarding of modified responses continues the process of bringing about a decrement in the strength of the more involuntary stuttering behavior. Stutterers begin to be able to modify their speech more effectively.

Building New Psychomotor Speech Patterns and Improving Speech Skills

Stuttering may be defined in part as unadaptive speech rigidity (Gregory, 1980). In its highly rigid nature, stuttering is analogous to most unadaptive patterns of behavior. As anxiety about stuttering diminishes and as stutterers become more able to cope with stuttering due to the analysis and modification activity just described, they can progress to building increased flexibility by practicing speech skills. They can learn variations in rate, loudness, inflection, phrasing, pause time, etc. The significance of this activity is that it increases even further the stutterer's positive expectations about speaking. The attitude we aim for is that a person who stutters can be a good speaker. But of course the person who is successful with the entire therapeutic strategy will communicate better and better, stutter less and less, and be steadily more comfortable and effective as a speaker.

In practice, although these four areas of therapy are related, two of them — changing attitude and diminishing bodily tension through the use of relaxation exercises — are usually stressed first, followed by analyzing and modifying speech and building speech skills. It is apparent how the stutter-more-fluently and the speak-more-fluently models are combined. The stutter-more-fluently model is emphasized first; however, therapy aimed toward desensitization of stuttering continues as increased fluency occurs and as new psychomotor speech patterns are practiced. Finally, bearing in mind the central point of this study, we should realize that one stutterer may need considerable help in reevaluating his perception of himself, whereas another will have more need for therapy concentrating on modifying her stuttering and improving her speech.Reference should be made to the interest in the use of drugs (sedatives, stimulants, and tranquilizers) as an adjunct to the usual procedure in stuttering therapy. Examples of research studies are the ones by Kent and Williams (1959), Burr and Mullendore (1960), and Aron (1965). As might be expected, it is a general observation that the tranquilizers diminish the severity of stuttering more than they affect frequency and that a calming effect may be useful when prominent neurotic elements are present. Again, different stutterers may be helped by different drugs. Clinicians must get to know the unique needs of their clients by establishing a relationship in which the clinician comes across as sincerely interested in and wanting to understand the client.

Therapy for More Confirmed Elementary School-Age Stutterers

With the age group from 6 or 7 to around 14 years of age, it is difficult to evaluate awareness, the consistency of avoidance and inhibitory tendencies, and the child's self-image as a person with a speech problem. Consequently, the issue of stutter-more-fluently vs. speak-more-fluently fades in importance. Gregory (1979b) concluded that there is essential agreement among clinicians such as Bloodstein, Cooper, Gregory, Perkins, Ryan, Van Riper, Webster, and Williams (representing differing basic beliefs about stuttering) that procedures should be used to enhance children's confidence in their ability to speak easily and enjoy communication. In recent years, Adams (1984), Costello (1984), and Shine (1984) have recommended sequences of procedures for improving the school-age child's fluency. Analysis of stuttering behavior is, in general, viewed as counterproductive, as would be true of therapy for a preschool child. Gregory (1973b, 1984a) and Williams (1971, 1979) have emphasized that work with this age group must be concrete and closely related to specific experience, both in terms of speech modifications and the development of appropriate attitudes. The approaches described below illustrate concrete, organized approaches to speech modification (Gregory, 1984a).

A *less specific approach* is used first in which the clinician models an easier, more relaxed approach with smooth movement (ERA-SM) beginning with words, then phrases, and gradually working up to longer, more complex utterances. ERA-SM involves a somewhat slower phonetic rate and transition between sounds at the *beginning* of a word or a phrase. A smooth transition from sound to sound and word to word is practiced. It may be necessary to use a somewhat slower general speech rate at first, but it is important to keep the change of rate and prosody to a minimum. Of course, if a rate problem or a cluttering element is present, appropriate modifications are made. Pausing, the resistance of time pressure in talking, and general relaxation are a part of the program. We point out to the child that an increased feeling of bodily relaxation is being carried over into the coordinated movements of exhalation, phonation, and articulation. The following are examples of steps in the program.

1. Using a tape recorder, the clinician models speech behavior that is "more relaxed and easy." The child is shown how "to make easy, relaxed smooth movements into words and between words." The tape is played back, and the child and clinician listen to the clinician's speech.

2. The clinician and child tape a choral reading. A relaxed manner of speaking with smooth movements into and between words is emphasized as was modeled by the clinician. The child and clinician listen to their speech on the tape. The microphone may be placed nearer to the child after several trials.

3. The clinician and child tape a choral reading again. Clinician drops out and joins the child again after a few words, a sentence, and so forth. The child is rewarded for imitating "more easy, relaxed speech with smooth movement."

4. The child is rewarded for "more easy, relaxed speech" as he or she reads or speaks spontaneously at the word, phrase, or sentence level, or as the child reads and speaks more extensively. Activities at varying levels may include answering short questions, describing objects, pictures, and events, and conversational speaking. The clinician arranges steps of increasing difficulty with great care. The child is taught self-monitoring and self-evaluation.

5. More and more emphasis is placed on exploration and experimentation with psychomotor speech responses, emphasizing relaxed initiation, smooth transitions between words, loudness and pitch variation, phrasing, and so forth.

A *more specific approach* is employed if the cues associated with stuttering on particular sounds and words are of the strength that stuttering still occurs. The following steps may be used:

1. The clinician feigns the introduction of tension in his or her speech to produce syllable repetitions, sound prolongations, vocal tension, etc. The child imitates some of these feigned behaviors.

2. The clinician models the modification of this feigned stuttering by, for example, slowing a repetition, shortening a prolongation, or easing the tension in the initiation of a vowel. The child does the same, imitating the feigned behaviors and modifications modeled by the clinician.

3. Following the clinician's model, the child imitates the actual difficulty he or she is having and then experiments with ways of modifying the tension and fragmentation involved.

4. This modification is finally evolved into ERA-SM.

5. Voluntary disfluency may be modeled and taught if the child is unduly sensitive about disfluency. Children need to understand that some disfluency is a normal aspect of speech.

This more specific approach is used only to the extent needed, and it varies depending on the outcome of using the less specific approach. In my experience some children will need this kind of extensive work on only a few sounds, others on several words, and a few on many aspects of speech production.

When the child has gained considerable self-confidence in speaking, I have found it important to reinforce this activity by role playing situations, reading poetry, and giving talks.

Children's attitudes are dealt with in two ways: (1) by talking about speech production in concrete terms and making analogies between therapy exercises and activities of interest to children, such as learning a skill in a sport or building a model car or airplane, and (2) being a good listener and adopting a supportive, understanding attitude toward the child. The child should be helped to explore an expressed concern using concrete behavioral terminology.

The same type of in-depth speech and language evaluation as previously described is carried out with this age group, and the therapy emphasizes different factors depending on need. Some school children who stutter have concomitant language problems, articulation problems, below-average motor control of speech structures, or communicative and interpersonal stress factors to be considered. Parents are taught relaxation procedures, and just like their children, they learn to carry the more relaxed feeling over into easy, relaxed approaches and smooth movements in their speech. From the clinician's model the parents also learn how to modify interactive behaviors and when to reinforce their children's modified speech.

Transfer and Maintenance

With all of the developmental stages and age groups discussed, the increasing of fluency and the decreasing of stuttering in the clinical or school therapy situation is not particularly difficult. The challenge for the clinician is in bringing about the change in such a way that it is transferred to real-life situations and that it persists over time. Both of these objectives require specific attention. The following statements highlight comments that have been made in the literature during the last 15 years on the topics of transfer and maintenance:

1. Continuing the process of transfer is probably important in maintenance, and maintaining gains enhances transfer.

2. As therapy progresses, activities should be planned to enable a child or an adult to emit changed speech in progressively more natural environmental situations. With a preschool child, the parents take part in therapy, acquiring changes in their way of interacting with the child as modeled by the clinician. In the normal progression, the parents are given assignments to do at home that reinforce what they have done at the clinic. With children between the ages of 6 or 7 and 12 or 13, the parents can participate in the same way as with younger children, but they can also learn how to reinforce the child for speech change. The clinician also needs to work with a child's teachers so that they can understand the child's therapy and be supportive. Transfer activities in the classroom can be planned. Adult stutterers and their clinicians can agree upon a hierarchy of speaking situations from easiest to most difficult. The objective of transferring speech changes utilizing the hierarchy begins with role playing in the therapy situation and then attempting changes in actual situations.

3. The stutterer's attitudes are important in terms of effective transfer and maintenance. Stutterers should understand the process nature of change (rapid change does not necessarily mean lasting change). They should realize that through therapy they can gain insight into their own feelings and thoughts that will facilitate transfer and maintenance, and that it takes time to integrate changes in attitude and behavior.

4. Therapy should begin with fairly intensive work and gradually taper off to less intensive and finally infrequent, depending on what is desirable for each individual.

5. Activitives directed toward the maintenance of therapeutic change include scheduled clinic visits and a home program. Clinic visits take a variety of forms, including evening visits, refresher weekends, and booster sessions lasting several days. Home programs include daily reviews, speech assignments, and daily speech recordings. Children are brought into the clinic for

rechecks, and the clinician keeps in touch with the parents by telephone and by home visits.

The reader should see Shames and Florance (1980), Boberg (1981), and Fraser-Gruss (1983) for further discussion of the theory and procedures of transfer and maintenance.

Recent Developments and Future Trends

In revising this book, first published in 1973, I have realized in a striking way just what developments have taken place during the last 10 years. And having been a professional speech-language pathologist specializing in stuttering for 30 years, I began to engage in some speculation about the future. Therefore, this last section will list some major developments and future prospects in this field.

Recent developments include the following:

1. We can make much better decisions about when to be concerned about a child's disfluency.
2. We have gained a better understanding of motor and linguistic factors related to stuttering and how to manage these as an integral part of therapy.
3. Progress has been made in assessing more objectively parent-child interaction factors that contribute to increased disfluency and stuttering in a child.
4. Through multidisciplinary clinics with clinical psychologists and psychiatrists, we deal more effectively with psychosocial factors related to stuttering problems.
5. Clinicians have learned to utilize behavior modification concepts (including modeling procedures) more systematically and effectively in changing the behavior of children who stutter, their parents, and adult stutterers.
6. The controversy between the advocates of the stutter-more-fluently approach and the speak-more-fluently approach has been clarified, and many clinicians are integrating the two.
7. We have faced up to the definite need for planned transfer and maintenance procedures with children and adults.
8. Increased measurement of therapeutic progress and outcome, in terms of speech and attitude changes (the former more effectively than the latter), has resulted in more efficient and effective therapy.

Future prospects are as follows:

1. Additional basic research about the nature of fluency, disfluency, and stuttering will add to our knowledge. More in-depth studies of individual cases

will be done in clinics and research laboratories. Variables will be measured more precisely.

2. Differential evaluation and treatment will become more precise. Yet we will continue to understand that experienced clinicians recognize important characteristics of clinical cases that cannot be quantified.

3. More research should pursue the difficult issue of interaction between subject (child or adult) variables and environmental variables in the development or maintenance of stuttering.

4. More clinicians will specialize in certain speech and language disorders including stuttering. They will go to centers where effective therapy is being done for postgraduate observation and instruction.

5. Children who stutter, their parents, and adult stutterers will be referred to clinicians who have proven competence in the area of fluency.

6. Follow-up interviews of stutterers and, in the case of children, follow-up interviews of parents will provide valuable insight into the therapy process as viewed by those who have experienced the problem.

References

Adams, M. (1984). The young stutterer: Diagnosis, treatment, and assessment of progress. In W. Perkins (Ed.), *Stuttering disorders* (pp. 41–56). New York: Theime–Stratton.

Ainsworth, S., & Fraser–Gruss, J. (1977). *If your child stutters: A guide for parents.* Memphis: Speech Foundation of America.

Andrews, G., et al. (1983). Stuttering: A review of research findings and theories circa 1982. *Journal of Speech and Hearing Disorders, 48,* 226–246.

Andrews, G., & Harris, M. (1964). *The syndrome of stuttering.* Spastics Society Medical Education and Information Unit. London: Levenham Press.

Arnold, G. E. (1965). Present concepts of etiologic factors. In *Studies in tachyphemia* (pp. 3–23). New York: Speech Rehabilitation Institute.

Aron, M. L. (1965). The effects of the combination of trifluoperazine and amylobarbitone on adult stutterers. *Medical Proceedings of the South African Journal for the Advancement of Medical Science, 11,* 227–233.

Bellak, L. (1954). *The thematic apperception test and children's apperception test in clinical use.* New York: Grune and Stratton.

Bender, L. (1946). *Instructions for use of the visual motor gestalt test.* New York: American Orthopsychiatric Association.

Berry, M. F. (1938). Developmental history of stuttering children. *Journal of Pediatrics, 12,* 209–217.

Berry, M. F., & Eisenson, J. (1956). *Speech disorders.* New York: Appleton–Century–Crofts.

Blaesing, L. (1982). A multidisciplinary approach to individualized treatment of stuttering. *Journal of Fluency Disorders, 7,* 203–218.

Blood, G. W., & Seider, R. (1981). The concomitant problems of young stutterers. *Journal of Speech and Hearing Disorders, 46,* 31–33.

Bloodstein, O. (1958). Stuttering as an anticipatory struggle reaction. In J. Eisenson (Ed.), *Stuttering: A symposium* (pp. 3–69). New York: Harper & Row.

Bloodstein, O. (1969). *A handbook on stuttering.* Chicago: National Easter Seal Society.

Bloodstein, O. (1975). Stuttering as tension and fragmentation. In J. Eisenson (Ed.), *Stuttering: A second symposium.* New York: Harper & Row.

Bloodstein, O. (1981). *A handbook on stuttering* (rev. ed.). Chicago: National Easter Seal Society.

Bloodstein, O., Jaeger, W., & Tureen, J. (1952). A study of the diagnosis of stuttering by parents of stutterers and non-stutterers. *Journal of Speech and Hearing Disorders, 17,* 308–315.

Bloodstein, O., & Gantwerk, B. (1967). Grammatical function in relation to stuttering in young children. *Journal of Speech and Hearing Research, 10*, 786–789.

Boberg, E. (Ed.). (1981). *Maintenance of fluency*. New York: Elsevier.

Boehmler, R. M. (1958). Listener responses to non-fluencies. *Journal of Speech and Hearing Research, 1*, 132–141.

Branscom, M. E., Hughes, J., & Oxtoby, E. T. (1955). Studies of nonfluency in the speech of preschool children. In W. Johnson (Ed.), *Stuttering in children and adults* (pp. 157–180). Minneapolis: University of Minnesota Press.

Brown, S. F. (1938). A further study of stuttering in relation to various speech sounds. *Quarterly Journal of Speech, 24*, 390–397.

Brownell, W. (1973). *The relationship of sex, social class, and verbal planning to the disfluencies produced by non-stuttering preschool children*. Unpublished doctoral dissertation, State University of New York at Buffalo.

Brutten, E. J., & Shoemaker, D. J. (1967). *The modification of stuttering*. Englewood Cliffs, NJ: Prentice-Hall.

Burr, H. G., & Mullendore, J. M. (1960). Recent investigations of tranquilizers and stuttering. *Journal of Speech and Hearing Disorders, 25*, 33–337.

Carrow, E. (1974). *Carrow Test of Auditory Comprehension for Language. Carrow Elicited Language Inventory*. Austin, TX: Learning Concepts.

Cheasman, C. (1983). Therapy for adults: An evaluation of current techniques for establishing fluency. In P. Dalton (Ed.), *Approaches to the treatment of stuttering*. London: Croom Helm.

Conture, E. (1984). *Letting information cloud our judgment about children who stutter*. Lecture presented at the 1984 Diamond Conference, Temple University, Philadelphia.

Cooper. E. B. (1972). Recovery from stuttering in a junior and senior high school population. *Journal of Speech and Hearing Research, 15*, 632–638.

Cooper, E. B. (1973). The development of a stuttering chronicity prediction checklist for school-aged stutterers: A research inventory for clinicians. *Journal of Speech and Hearing Research, 38*, 215–223.

Cooper, E. B. (1979). Intervention procedures for the young stutterer. In H. Gregory (Ed.), *Controversies about stuttering therapy* (pp. 63–69). Austin, TX: PRO-ED.

Costello, J. (1984). Operant conditioning and the treatment of stuttering. In W. Perkins (Ed.), *Stuttering disorders* (pp. 107–127). New York: Theime-Stratton.

Curry, F. K. W., & Gregory, H. (1969). The performance of stutterers on dichotic listening tasks thought to reflect cerebral dominance. *Journal of Speech and Hearing Research, 12*, 73–82.

Dalton, P. (1983). Maintenance of change; Towards the integration of behavioural and psychological procedures. In P. Dalton (Ed.), *Approaches to the treatment of stuttering* (pp. 163–184). London: Croom Helm.

Darley, F. L. (1955). The relationship of parental attitudes and adjustments to the development of stuttering. In W. Johnson (Ed.), *Stuttering in children and adults* (pp. 74–153). Minneapolis: University of Minnesota Press.

Davis, D. M. (1939). The relation of repetitions in the speech of young children to certain measures of language maturity and situational factors: Part I. *Journal of Speech Disorders, 4,* 303–318.

Decker, T., Healey, E., & Howe, S. (1982). Brainstem auditory electrical response characteristics of stutterers and non-stutters: A preliminary report. *Journal of Fluency Disorders, 7,* 385–401.

DeJoy, D. (1975). *An investigation of the frequency of nine individual types of disfluency and total disfluency in relation to age and syntactic maturity in nonstuttering males, three and one-half years of age and five years of age.* Unpublished doctoral dissertation, Northwestern University, Evanston, IL.

Doll, E. A. (1947a). *The Osretsky Test of Motor Proficiency.* Minneapolis: Educational Publishers, Inc.

Doll, E. A. (1947b). *Vineland Social Maturity Scale: Manual of directions.* Minneapolis: Educational Test Bureau.

Dollard, J., & Miller, N. E. (1950). *Personality and psychotherapy.* New York: McGraw-Hill.

Dunn, L. M. (1965). *Expanded manual: Peabody Picture Vocabulary Test.* Minneapolis: American Guidance Service.

Egland, G. O. (1955). Repetitions and prolongations in the speech of stuttering and nonstuttering children. In W. Johnson (Ed.), *Stuttering in children and adults* (pp. 181–188). Minneapolis: University of Minnesota Press.

Eisenson, J. (1965). Speech disorders. In B. Wolman (Ed.), *Handbook of clinical psychology* (pp. 765–784). New York: McGraw-Hill.

Eisenson, J., & Winslow, C. N. (1938). The perseverating tendency in stutterers in a perceptual function. *Journal of Speech Disorders, 3,* 195–198.

Fox, D. R. (1966). Electroencephalographic analysis during stuttering and nonstuttering. *Journal of Speech and Hearing Research, 9,* 488–497.

Fraser-Gruss, J. (Ed.). (1981). *Counseling stutterers.* Memphis, TN: Speech Foundation of America.

Fraser-Gruss, J. (Ed.). (1983). *Stuttering: Transfer and maintenance.* Memphis. TN: Speech Foundation of America.

Freund, H. (1966). *Psychopathology and the problems of stuttering.* Springfield, IL: Charles C. Thomas.

Gesell, A., & Amatruda, C. S. (1948). *Developmental diagnosis.* New York: Paul Hoeber.

Giolas, T. G., & Williams, D. E. (1958). Children's reaction to nonfluencies in adult speech. *Journal of Speech and Hearing Research, 1,* 86–93.

Glasner, P. J. (1949). Personality characteristics and emotional problems in stutterers under the age of five. *Journal of Speech and Hearing Disorders, 14,* 135–138.

Glasner, P. J. (1970). Developmental view. In J. Sheehan (Ed.), *Stuttering: Research and therapy.* New York: Harper & Row.

Goodstein, L. D. (1958). Functional speech disorders and personality: A survey of the research. *Journal of Speech and Hearing Research, 1,* 359–376.

Gottfred, K. (1979). *A longitudinal analysis of type and frequency of disfluency, related to communicative pressure and length of utterance, in children 24 to 36 months of age.* Unpublished doctoral dissertation, Northwestern University, Evanston, IL.

Graham, J. K. (1966). A neurologic and electroencephalographic study of adult stutterers and matched normal speakers [abstract]. *Speech Monographs, 33,* 290.

Gray, B., & England, G. (1969). Stuttering: The measurement of anxiety during reciprocal inhibition. In B. Gray & G. England (Eds.), *Stuttering and the conditioning therapies* (pp. 47–56). Monterey, CA: Monterey Institute for Speech and Hearing.

Gregory, H. (1968a). Applications of learning theory concepts in the management of stuttering. In H. Gregory (Ed.), *Learning theory and stuttering therapy* (pp. 107–128). Evanston, IL: Northwestern University Press.

Gregory, H. (1968b). Summary, conclusions, implications. In H. Gregory (Ed.), *Learning theory and stuttering therapy* (pp. 129–148). Evanston, IL: Northwestern University Press.

Gregory, H. (1973a). Modeling procedure in the treatment of elementary school age children who stutter. *Journal of Fluency Disorders, 1,* 58–63.

Gregory, H. (1973b). *Stuttering: Differential evaluation and therapy.* Indianapolis: Bobbs-Merrill.

Gregory, H. (1979a). Controversial issues: Statement and review of the literature. In H. Gregory (Ed.), *Controversies about stuttering therapy* (pp. 1–62). Austin, TX: PRO-ED.

Gregory, H. (1979b). Controversial issues: Analysis and current status. In H. Gregory (Ed.), *Controversies about stuttering therapy* (pp. 269–292). Austin, TX: PRO-ED.

Gregory, H. (1980). Contemporary issues in stuttering therapy. *Journal of Fluency Disorders, 5,* 291–302.

Gregory, H. (1984a). Prevention of stuttering and the management of early developmental stages. In R. Curlee & W. Perkins (Eds.), *Nature and treatment of stuttering* (pp. 335–355). San Diego, CA: College Hill Press.

Gregory, H. (Ed.). (1984b). *Stuttering therapy: Prevention and intervention with children.* Memphis, TN: Speech Foundation of America.

Gregory, H. (1985). Environmental modifications. In G. Shames & H. Rubin (Eds.), *Stuttering: Then and now.* Columbus, OH: Charles Merrill.

Gregory, H., & Hill, D. (1980). Stuttering therapy for children. In W. Perkins (Ed.), *Strategies in stuttering therapy.* New York: Theime-Stratton.

Gregory, H., & Hill, D. (1984). Stuttering therapy for children. In W. Perkins (Ed.), *Stuttering disorders.* New York: Theime-Stratton.

Gregory, H., & Mangan, J. (1982). Auditory processes in stutterers. In N. Lass (Ed.), *Speech and language: Advances in basic research and practice* (pp. 71–103). New York: Academic Press.

Guitar, B., & Peters, T. (1980). *Stuttering: An integration of contemporary therapies.* Memphis TN: Speech Foundation of America.

Hall, J. W., & Jerger, J. (1978). Central auditory function in stutterers. *Journal of Speech and Hearing Research, 21,* 324–337.

Hall, P. K. (1977). The occurrence of disfluencies in language-disordered children. *Journal of Speech and Hearing Disorders, 42*, 364–369.

Haynes, W., & Hood, S. (1977). Disfluency changes in children as a function of the systematic modification of linguistic complexity. *Journal of Communicative Disorders, 11*, 79–93.

Helmreich, H., & Bloodstein, O. (1973). The grammatical factor in childhood disfluency in relation to the continuity hypothesis. *Journal of Speech and Hearing Research, 16*, 731–738.

Holland, A. (1967). Some applications of behavioral principles to clinical speech problems. *Journal of Speech and Hearing Disorders, 32*, 11–18.

Howie, P. M. (1981). A twin investigation of the etiology of stuttering. *Journal of Speech and Hearing Research, 24*, 317–321.

Ingham, R. (1984). Towards a therapy assessment procedure for treating stuttering in children. In H. Gregory (Ed.), *Stuttering: Intervention with children*. Memphis, TN: Speech Foundation of America.

Jacobson, E. (1938). *Progressive relaxation*. Chicago: University of Chicago Press.

Johnson, W., et al. (1959). *The onset of stuttering*. Minneapolis: University of Minnesota Press.

Johnson, W. (1967). Stuttering. In W. Johnson & D. Moeller (Eds.), *Speech-handicapped school children*. New York: Harper & Row.

Johnson, W. (Ed.). (1955). *Stuttering in children and adults*. Minneapolis: University of Minnesota Press.

Johnston, W., et al. (1942). A study of the onset and development of stuttering. *Journal of Speech Disorders, 7*, 251–257.

Johnson, W., Darley, F. L., & Spriestersbach, D. C. (1963). *Diagnostic methods in speech pathology*. New York: Harper & Row.

Kasprisin, A. (1970, Nov.). *Implications of parental verbal behavior for stuttering therapy with children*. Paper presented at the meeting of the American Speech and Hearing Association, New York.

Kasprisin-Burrelli, A., Egolf, D., & Shames, G. (1972). A comparison of parental verbal behavior with stuttering and nonstuttering children. *Journal of Communication Disorders, 5*, 335–346.

Kent, L. R., & Williams, D. E. (1959). Use of meprobamate as an adjunct to stuttering therapy. *Journal of Speech and Hearing Disorders, 24*, 64–69.

Kidd, K. K. (1980). Genetic models of stuttering. *Journal of Fluency Disorders, 5*, 187–201.

Kidd, K. K. (1983). Recent progress on the genetics of stuttering. In C. Ludlow & J. Cooper (Eds.), *Genetic aspects of speech and language disorders*. New York: Academic Press.

Kimura, D. (1967). Functional asymmetry of the brain in dichotic listening. *Cortex, 3*, 163–178.

Kirk, S. A., McCarthy, J. J., & Kirk, W. D. (1968). *Examiner's manual: Illinois Test of Psycholinguistic Abilities*. Urbana, IL: University of Illinois Press.

Lee, L. (1969). *Northwestern Syntax Screening Test*. Evanston, IL: Northwestern University Press.

Lemert, E. M. (1953). Some Indians who stutter. *Journal of Speech and Hearing Disorders, 18,* 168–174.

Lemert, E. M. (1962). Stuttering and social structure in two Pacific societies. *Journal of Speech and Hearing Disorders, 27,* 3–10.

Luchsinger, R., & Landolt, H.L. (1951). Elektroenzephalographische Untersuchungen bei Stotterern mit und ohne Polterkomponente [Electroencephalographic study of stutterers with and without cluttering]. *Folia Phoniatrica, 3,* 135–150.

Luper, H. L. (1968). An appraisal of learning theory concepts in understanding and treating stuttering in children. In H. Gregory (Ed.), *Learning theory and stuttering therapy* (pp. 84–106). Evanston, IL: Northwestern University Press.

Luper, H. L., & Mulder, R. L. (1964). *Stuttering: Therapy for children*. Englewood Cliffs, NJ: Prentice-Hall.

Luper, H., & Cross, D. E. (1978, Nov.). *Relation between finger reaction time and voice reaction time in stuttering and non-stuttering children and adults*. Paper presented at the annual convention of the American Speech-Language-Hearing Association, San Francisco.

Merits-Patterson, R., & Reed, C. (1981). Disfluencies in the speech of language-delayed children. *Journal of Speech and Hearing Research, 24,* 55–58.

Miller, N. E. (1944). Experimental studies of conflict. In J. McV. Hunt (Ed.), *Personality and the behavior disorders* (pp. 344–453). New York: Ronald Press.

Moncur, J. P. (1952). Parental domination in stuttering. *Journal of Speech and Hearing Disorders, 17,* 115–165.

Moore, W. H., & Haynes, W. O. (1980). Alpha hemispheric asymmetry and stuttering: Some support for a segmentation dysfunction hypothesis. *Journal of Speech and Hearing Research, 23,* 229–247.

Moore, W. H., & Lorendo, L. C. (1980). Hemispheric alpha asymmetries of stuttering and non-stuttering males and females for words of high or low imagery. *Journal of Fluency Disorders, 5,* 11–26.

Mordecai, D. (1979). *An investigation of the communicative styles of mothers and fathers of stuttering versus nonstuttering preschool children during a triadic interaction*. Unpublished doctoral dissertation, Northwestern University, Evanston, IL.

Morgenstern, J. J. (1956). Socio-economic factors in stuttering. *Journal of Speech and Hearing Disorders, 21,* 25–33.

Nelson, L. (1984). Language formulation related to disfluency and stuttering. In H. Gregory (Ed.), *Stuttering therapy: Prevention and intervention with children* (pp. 43–62). Memphis, TN: Speech Foundation of America.

Oxtoby, E. (1943). *A quantitative study of the repetitions in the speech of three-year-old children*. Unpublished master's thesis, University of Iowa, Iowa City.

Perkins, W. (1979). From psychoanalysis to discoordination. In H. Gregory (Ed.), *Controversies about stuttering therapy* (pp. 97–128). Austin, TX: PRO-ED.

Perkins, W. (1983). The problem of definition: Commentary on "stuttering." *Journal of Speech and Hearing Disorders, 48,* 246–249.

Pratt, J. E. (1972). *Comparison of linguistic perception and production in preschool stutterers and non-stutterers.* Unpublished doctoral dissertation, University of Illinois, Urbana-Champaign.

Quinn, P. T. (1972). Stuttering, cerebral dominance, and the dichotic word test. *Medical Journal of Australia, 2,* 639–643.

Reich, A., Till, J., & Goldsmith, H. (1981). Laryngeal and manual reaction times of stuttering and non-stuttering adults. *Journal of Speech and Hearing Research, 24,* 192–196.

Riley, G., & Riley, J. (1979). A component model for diagnosing and treating children who stutter. *Journal of Fluency Disorders, 4,* 279–293.

Riley, G., & Riley, J. (1980). Motoric and linguistic variables among children who stutter: A factor analysis. *Journal of Speech and Hearing Disorders, 45,* 504–514.

Riley, G., & Riley, J. (1983). Evaluation as a basis for intervention. In D. Prins & R. Ingham (Eds.), *Treatment of stuttering in early childhood* (pp. 43–67). San Diego: College Hill Press.

Ryan, B. (1974). *Programmed therapy for stuttering in children and adults.* Springfield, IL: Charles C. Thomas.

Ryan, B. (1979). Stuttering therapy in a framework of operant conditioning and programmed learning. In H. Gregory (Ed.), *Controversies about stuttering therapy* (pp. 129–176). Austin, TX: PRO-ED.

Schindler, M. D. (1955). A study of educational adjustments of stuttering and non-stuttering children. In W. Johnson (Ed.), *Stuttering in children and adults* (pp. 348–357). Minneapolis: University of Minnesota Press.

Schwartz, R. G. (1983). Diagnosis of speech sound disorders in children. In I. J. Meitus & B. Weinberg (Eds.), *Diagnosis in speech-language pathology* (pp. 113–149). Austin, TX: PRO-ED.

Shames, G. H., & Sherrick, C. E., Jr., (1963). A discussion of non-fluency and stuttering as operant behavior. *Journal of Speech and Hearing Disorders, 28,* 3–18.

Shames, G., & Florance, C. (1980). *Stutter-free speech.* Columbus, OH: Charles Merrill.

Sheehan, J. G. (1953). Theory and treatment of stuttering as an approach-avoidance conflict. *Journal of Psychology, 36,* 27–49.

Sheehan, J. G. (1958a). Conflict theory of stuttering. In J. Eisenson (Ed.), *Stuttering: A symposium* (pp. 121–166). New York: Harper & Row.

Sheehan, J. G. (1958b). Projective studies of stuttering. *Journal of Speech and Hearing Disorders, 23,* 18–25.

Sheehan, J. G. (1968). Stuttering as self-role conflict. In H. H. Gregory (Ed.), *Learning theory and stuttering therapy* (pp. 72–83). Evanston, IL: Northwestern University Press.

Sheehan, J. G. (1970). *Stuttering: Research and therapy.* New York: Harper & Row.

Sheehan, J. G. (1975). Conflict theory and avoidance-reduction therapy. In J. Eisenson (Ed.), *Stuttering: A second symposium* (pp. 97–198). New York: Harper & Row.

Sheehan, J. G., & Martyn, M. M. (1966). Spontaneous recovery from stuttering. *Journal of Speech and Hearing Research, 9,* 121–135.

Sheehan, J. G., & Martyn, M. M. (1970). Stuttering and its disappearance. *Journal of Speech and Hearing Research, 13*, 279–287.

Sheehan, J. G., & Costley, M. S. (1977). A reexamination of the role of heredity in stuttering. *Journal of Speech and Hearing Disorders, 42*, 47–59.

Sheehan, J. G., & Sheehan, V. (1984). Avoidance-reduction therapy: A response suppression hypothesis. In W. Perkins (Ed.), *Stuttering disorders*. New York: Theime-Stratton.

Shine, R. (1984). Assessment of fluency training with the young stutterer. In M. Peins (Ed.), *Contemporary approaches in stuttering therapy* (pp. 173–216). Boston: Little Brown.

Silverman, E. (1972). Generality of disfluency data collected from preschoolers. *Journal of Speech and Hearing Research, 15*, 84–92.

Silverman, E. (1973). The influence of preschoolers' speech usage on their disfluency frequency. *Journal of Speech and Hearing Research, 16*, 474–481.

Skinner, B. F. (1953). *Science and human behavior*. New York: Macmillan.

Snidecor, J. C. (1947). Why the Indian does not stutter. *Quarterly Journal of Speech, 33*, 493–495.

Sommers, R., Brady, W., & Moore, W. (1975). Dichotic ear preference of stuttering children and adults. *Perceptual and Motor Skills, 41*, 931–938.

Starkweather, C. W. (1982). Stuttering and laryngeal behavior: A review. *ASHA Monographs, 21*. Rockville, MD: American Speech-Language-Hearing Association.

Stewart, J. L. (1960). The problem of stuttering in certain North American Indian societies. *Journal of Speech and Hearing Disorders Monograph Supplement, 6*.

Stromsta, C. (1959). Experimental blockage of phonation by distorted sidetone. *Journal of Speech and Hearing Research, 2*, 286–301.

Sussman, H., & MacNeilage, P. (1975). Studies of hemispheric specialization for speech production. *Brain and Language, 2*, 131–151.

Taylor, I. K. (1966). The properties of stuttered words. *Journal of Verbal Learning and Verbal Behavior, 5*, 112–118.

Tomatis, A. (1956). Relations entre l'audition et la phonation. *Extroit des Annales des Teleco·nmunications*, vol. 2.

Toscher, M. M., & Rupp, R. R. (1978). A study of the central auditory processes in stutterers using the synthetic sentence identification (SSI) test battery. *Journal of Speech and Hearing Research, 21*, 779–792.

Travis, L. E. (1931). *Speech pathology*. New York: Appleton-Century.

Travis, L. E. (1957). The unspeakable feelings of people, with special reference to stuttering. In L. E. Travis (Ed.), *Handbook of speech pathology* (pp. 916–946). New York: Appleton-Century-Crofts.

Van Riper, C. (1947, 1954, 1963). *Speech correction: Principles and methods*. 2nd, 3rd, and 4th eds. Englewood Cliffs, NJ: Prentice-Hall.

Van Riper, C. (1973). *The treatment of stuttering*. Englewood Cliffs, NJ: Prentice-Hall.

Van Riper, C. (1982). *The nature of stuttering*. Englewood Cliffs, NJ: Prentice-Hall.

Voelker, C. (1944). A preliminary investigation for a normative study of disfluency: A critical index to the severity of stuttering. *American Journal of Orthopsychiatry, 14*, 285–294.

Wall, M., & Myers, F. (Eds.). (1984). *Clinical management of childhood stuttering.* Austin, TX: PRO-ED.

Weiss, D. A. (1964). *Cluttering.* Englewood Cliffs, NJ: Prentice-Hall.

Wexler, K., & Mysak, E. (1982). Disfluency characteristics of 2-, 4-, and 6-year-old males. *Journal of Fluency Disorders, 7*, 37–46.

Williams, D. E. (1971). Stuttering therapy for children. In L. E. Travis (Ed.), *Handbook of speech pathology* (pp. 1073–1093). New York: Appleton-Century-Crofts.

Williams, D. E. (1979). A perspective on approaches to stuttering therapy. In H. Gregory (Ed.), *Controversies about stuttering therapy* (pp. 241–268). Austin, TX: PRO-ED.

Williams, D. E., & Kent, L. R. (1958). Listener evaluations of speech interruptions. *Journal of Speech and Hearing Research, 12*, 308–318.

Wingate, M. E. (1966). Prosody in stuttering adaptation. *Journal of Speech and Hearing Research, 9*, 550–556.

Wingate, M. E. (1967). Stuttering and word length. *Journal of Speech and Hearing Research, 10*, 146–152.

Wingate, M. E. (1971). Phonetic ability in stuttering. *Journal of Speech and Hearing Research, 14*, 189–194.

Wischner, G. J. (1950). Stuttering behavior and learning: A preliminary theoretical formulation. *Journal of Speech and Hearing Disorders, 15*, 324–335.

Wolpe, J. (1958). *Psychotherapy by reciprocal inhibition.* Stanford, CA: Stanford University Press.

Wyatt, G. (1969). *Language learning and communication disorders in children.* New York: The Free Press.

Yairi, E. (1981). Disfluencies of normally speaking two-year-old children. *Journal of Speech and Hearing Research, 24*, 490–495.

Yairi, E. (1982). Longitudinal studies of disfluencies in two-year-old children. *Journal of Speech and Hearing Research, 25*, 115–160.

Yairi, E. (1983). The onset of stuttering in two- and three-year-old children: A preliminary report. *Journal of Speech and Hearing Disorders, 48*, 171–177.

Hugo H. Gregory received his B.S., M.A., and Ph.D. degrees at Northwestern University, where he is now Professor and Head, Speech and Language Pathology, and Director of Stuttering Programs. He has edited two widely used books, *Learning Theory and Stuttering Therapy* and *Controversies about Stuttering Therapy*, has written numerous journal articles and chapters in books, and has contributed to several Speech Foundation of America publications on stuttering. He has lectured throughout the United States, in Canada, and in Europe. Professor Gregory has focused upon the definition of issues related to understanding the nature and treatment of stuttering as well as the practical clinical applications of research.